What's in This B[ook]

What To Do
For Healthy Teeth

Easy to Read • Easy to Use

Sadie S. Mestman, D.M.D.
Ariella D. Herman, Ph.D.

Institute for Healthcare Advancement
501 S. Idaho St., Suite 300
La Habra, California 90631
(800) 434-4633

Institute for Healthcare Advancement
501 S. Idaho Street, Suite 300
La Habra, California 90631

Library of Congress Cataloging-in-Publication Data
Mestman, Sadie S.
  What to do for healthy teeth : easy to read, easy to use / Sadie S.
Mestman, Ariella D. Herman.
      p. cm.
  Includes bibliographical references and index.
   ISBN 978-0-9720148-0-9 (pbk. : alk. paper)
  1. Teeth—Care and hygiene—Popular works. 2. Mouth—Care and
hygiene—Popular works. I. Herman, Ariella D. II. Title.
   RK61.M578 2004
   617.6'01—dc22

Printed in the United States of America
15 14 13   10 9 8 7
ISBN: 978-0-9720148-0-9

2004004252

To Our Readers

This book is written to help you take good care of your teeth and your children's teeth. It tells about how to take care of your teeth each day, and what to do in case of an emergency. There are pages that tell about eating right, taking care of your teeth when you are having a baby, and helping your children care for their teeth.

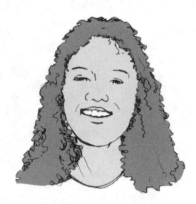

Healthy teeth are very important. Your teeth help you chew, speak, and smile. If you don't take care of your teeth you can get very sick. Use this book to know how to keep your teeth, mouth, and gums healthy.

Take a minute now and fill in the spaces inside the front cover of this book. Write in the phone numbers of your dentist, doctor, and drug store. Read the parts about emergencies now. That way you'll know what to do if you or someone in your family has an accident and hurts their teeth or mouth. Keep this book in a handy place so you can refer to it when you need it.

This book was written by a dentist and an educator, and read over by dentists and others who care for your mouth. They agree with the information in this book and feel it is helpful.

To Our Readers

This book does not take the place of going to the dentist. Everyone is different. So if you are having pain or have concerns about the advice in this book, talk to your dentist or doctor right away. Always do what your dentist or doctor says. And don't forget to visit your dentist every six months to be sure your teeth and gums are strong and healthy.

Safety Tips 1

Notes

_____

_____

_____

_____

_____

_____

_____

_____

_____

_____

_____

_____

_____

_____

Safety Tips

What are they?

Safety tips are things you can do to keep safe. These tips will help you keep your children safe too. If you keep your children safe, you can stop them from hurting their mouth, teeth and gums. Our teeth and gums help us talk and eat, so we need to take good care of them.

What can I do to keep my baby or small child safe?

Take care of teeth safely:

- Watch your children when they brush their teeth. Make sure kids three and older only use a pea-sized amount of toothpaste. Use only use a smear for kids under 3. Make sure they spit it out when they're done brushing. Don't let children swallow toothpaste or mouthwash.

- Don't let small children play with floss, toothbrushes, toothpaste or mouthwash. Children should only use a toothbrush at the sink. Never let them walk or run with a toothbrush in their hand or mouth.

- See page 67 to learn more about caring for children's teeth.

Safety Tips

Prevent choking:

- Give your baby a safe teething ring (See page 78). Do not give a teething ring with liquid inside it.

- If you give your baby a pacifier, make sure it is not cracked or torn. Your baby could swallow a piece of it and choke.

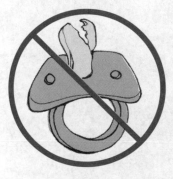

- Never put anything on a string around your child's neck. This includes a pacifier or teething ring. It could choke the child.

Prevent falling and accidents:

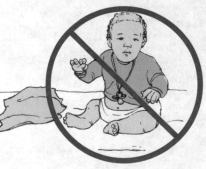

- Put your child in a car seat every time they ride in a car. These are special seats for babies and children that keep them safe in the car. Infants should be in a car seat that faces backward. They should be in this kind until they are 1 year old and weigh at least 20 pounds. Ask your nurse if you are not sure what kind of car seat your child needs.

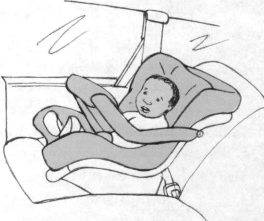

Safety Tips

- Always keep one hand on your child when they are on a changing table, bed, or chair. Your child could roll off.

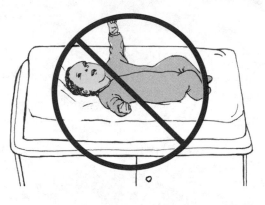

- Lower the crib mattress. That way your baby can't fall or climb out.

- Use child gates at the top and bottom of stairs.

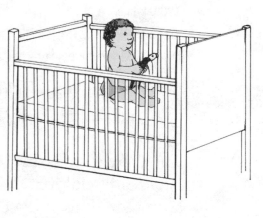

- Use a safety belt or infant seat if you put your child in a shopping cart. Never walk away from your child when using a cart.

- Don't let your child walk or run holding pointed things. Don't let them walk or run with a toothbrush in their mouth or in their hand.

- Make sure your child wears things to protect them when they play sports. This is important because your child could fall, get hit, or run into another child. For many sports, your child should wear a helmet or a mouth guard. (See page 103 to learn more about mouth guards.)

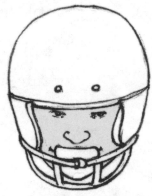

Safety Tips

Keep your child away from dangerous things:

- Do not leave curtain cords, blind cords, or electric cords where a child can reach them.

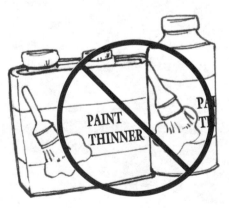

- Put socket covers on all outlets.

- Keep your child away from pet food. Never let your child go close to a pet when it is eating.

- Put safety locks on any cabinets that that your baby can reach. Make sure to lock cabinets where you keep medicines, cleaning supplies, or even toothpaste and mouthwash.

- Keep poisons where your baby or toddler can't see or touch them. Poisons are things that can hurt you- or even kill you- if you swallow them. All of these things could be poison:

  - Household cleaners
  - Paint
  - Paint thinner
  - Medicines
  - Health care and beauty products, like shampoo and makeup

The Mouth

Notes

_____

_____

_____

_____

_____

_____

_____

_____

_____

_____

_____

_____

_____

_____

The Mouth

What is it?

Your **mouth** is the part of your face you use to talk. You also use it to chew food and swallow.

What do I see?

In your mouth you will see teeth, gums, and a tongue.

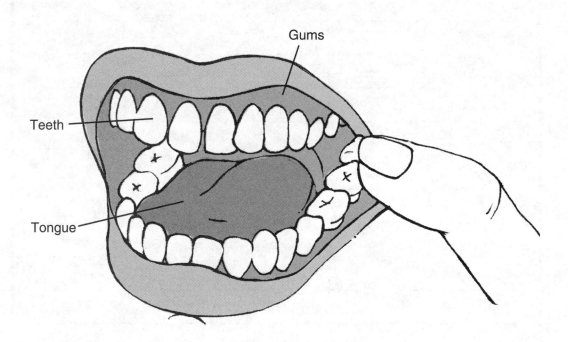

Teeth

What are they?

Teeth are the white, hard parts in your mouth. You use them to bite and chew food.

What do I see?

You can see 4 different kinds of teeth. They are different shapes, and you use them for different things.

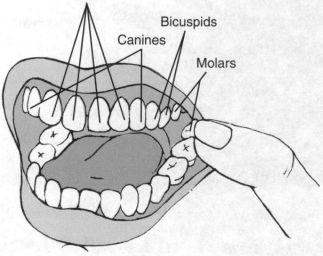

- **Incisors** are the front 8 teeth in your mouth. You have 4 on top and 4 on the bottom. You use them to bite into food and cut it.

- **Canines** are the teeth on each side of your front 4 teeth. They are also called **fang teeth** or **eye teeth**. You use them to rip and tear at tough food.

- **Bicuspids** are the 2 teeth behind the canines. You use these to crush food.

- **Molars** are the big, wide back teeth. You use them to crush and grind food into small bits so you can swallow it.

What can I do at home?

- Take good care of your teeth. Read this book to learn how to keep your teeth healthy.

- Use a soft toothbrush to brush your teeth 2 times a day with fluoride toothpaste. The most important time to brush is just before bedtime. (See page 30.)

- Eat foods that are good for you and your teeth. (See page 46.)

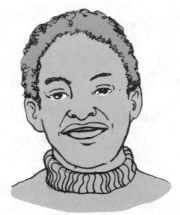

- Limit in-between-meal snacks.

- Use a mouth guard if you play a sport where you can hurt your teeth. (See page 103.)

- Don't eat too much food that has lots of sugar, like candy. Stay away from sweet and sticky foods that stay on your teeth, like gummy bears. (See page 46.)

- See a dentist every 6 months.

When should I call a dentist?

Call a dentist if:

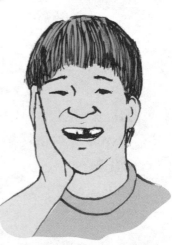

- you have pain in your mouth or teeth.

- you break, chip, or hurt your teeth.

See a dentist every 6 months, even if your teeth don't hurt. This is called a **checkup**.

What else should I know?

You have 2 sets of teeth in your life. Your first teeth are called **baby teeth**. They will fall out. Even though these teeth will fall out, you need to keep them healthy. After the baby teeth fall out, you get **adult teeth**. If you lose an adult tooth or it is pulled, you will not grow a new one in its place.

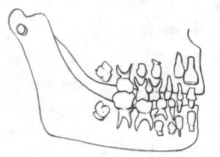

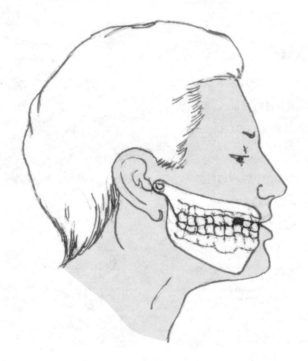

Gums

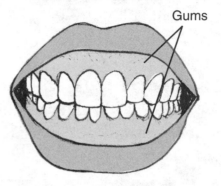

Gums

What are they?

Your **gums** are the pink part around your teeth.

What do I see?

Most gums are pink and fleshy. They also can be red or brown.

What can I do at home?

- Brush your teeth with a soft toothbrush 2 times a day with fluoride toothpaste.
- Floss between your teeth every day. When you floss, you clean between your teeth, and where your teeth touch your gums. You use string called **dental floss**. Learn more about flossing on page 36.

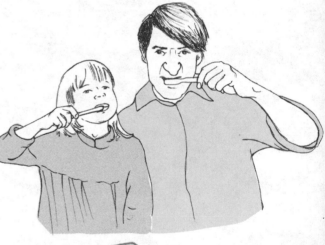

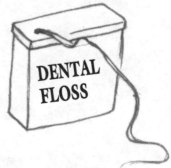

DENTAL FLOSS

Gums

When should I call a dentist?

Call a dentist if:

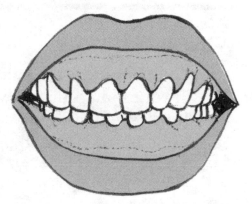

- your gums get big or puffy.
- your gums turn very red.
- your gums hurt.
- your gums bleed.

See the dentist for a checkup every 6 months. Do this even if your teeth and gums don't hurt.

What else should I know?

Healthy gums help hold your teeth in place. Keep your teeth and gums healthy to keep your body healthy.

Tongue

What is it?

Your **tongue** is the muscle in your mouth that moves. It helps you taste and swallow food. Your tongue also helps you talk.

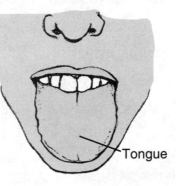
Tongue

What do I see?

The tongue looks different in everyone. Some tongues are smooth and pink. Some have deep grooves or cracks. Some look like a map with white marks.

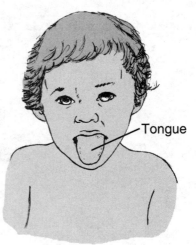
Tongue

What can I do at home?

- Keep your tongue clean and healthy, just like your teeth and gums.

- You can use a toothbrush or **tongue scraper** to clean your tongue. (See page 41.)

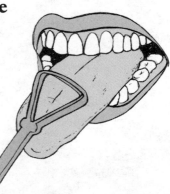

Tongue

When should I call a dentist?

Call a dentist if:

- you see red or white sores on your tongue. These can be on the top, bottom, or sides. Call your dentist even if the spots don't hurt.

- your tongue looks or feels different than usual.

- your tongue is swollen or hurts.

What else should I know?

Some people have a tongue that looks like a map of a country. It's called a **geographic tongue**. This won't hurt you; it just looks different. If you have this, your tongue will have red patches with white edges. The middle of your tongue may be more red than the sides.

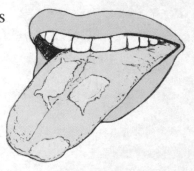

Some people have a tongue with grooves in it. This is called a **fissured tongue**. If you have this kind of tongue, it will look wrinkled. It will have deep and shallow grooves. This won't hurt you. You can't get it from someone else; some people are just born with it. It does not go away.

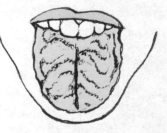

Your Teeth and Gums 3

Notes

_____

_____

_____

_____

_____

_____

_____

_____

_____

_____

_____

_____

_____

_____

Cavities

What is it?

A **cavity** (**kav**-uh-tee) is a hole in your tooth. It is also called **tooth decay** (di-**kay**). It's when your tooth rots.

What do I see?

A cavity may look whiter than the rest of your tooth. You may see a hole that is black, brown, or yellow. Sometimes you don't see anything, but you may have pain in a tooth. Your dentist may need a picture (**X-ray**) of the tooth to see the cavity.

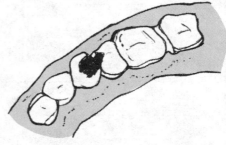

What can I do at home?

- Take good care of your teeth to prevent cavities.

  - Brush your teeth with a soft toothbrush two times a day with fluoride toothpaste. Brush when you wake up in the morning and before you go to bed at night. (See page 30.)

  - Floss between your teeth at least one time each day. (See page 36.)

  - See the dentist for a checkup every six months.

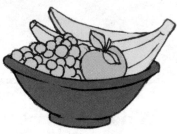

- Eat food that is good for you. Don't eat too many sugary foods like candy. Limit snacks between meals. (See page 46.)

- See your dentist if you think you have a cavity. You can't fix a cavity at home.

When should I call the dentist?

Call the dentist if:

- your tooth hurts when you eat things that are hot, cold, or sweet.

- your tooth hurts when you chew.

- food gets caught between your teeth, and you can't get it out.

- you see a hole in your tooth, or feel it with your tongue.

See the dentist every 6 months for a checkup. The dentist will check to make sure you don't have a cavity.

What else should I know?

Foods that have sugar cause cavities. When you have more sugar in your mouth, it helps more germs to grow. Germs in your mouth make acid that eats away at your teeth. This can make a hole in your tooth.

You can get a cavity at any age.

A cavity may not cause pain until it gets big. This is another reason to see your dentist every 6 months. Your dentist can fix a cavity early on, when it is still small.

Gingivitis

What is it?

Gingivitis (jin-ji-**vye**-tis) is when your gums get infected. You can get this if there is too much **plaque** around your teeth. (See page 24.)

What do I see?

Your gums may look red and puffy. They may bleed easily and feel tender or painful.

What can I do at home?

- If your gums are red, puffy, tender, or bleeding, call your dentist.

- Brush your teeth with a soft toothbrush 2 times a day and floss between your teeth 1 time a day. This can help prevent gingivitis.

- Take extra time to massage your gums with a soft toothbrush once a day. This cleans away the plaque that causes gingivitis. Wet your toothbrush with warm water and gently massage the area where the teeth and gums meet with the bristles. Your gums may feel a little tender, and you may notice some bleeding at first. Do not be afraid. It is important to be gentle when massaging your gums. If your gums keep bleeding, talk to your dentist.

- Rinse your mouth with salt water. Mix 1/2 glass of warm water with 1/2 teaspoon of salt. This helps the puffiness go away.

- Your gums will be better in about 2 weeks.

When should I call the dentist?

Call the dentist if:

- your gums bleed a lot and are very tender.
- your gums do not get better after 2 weeks.

See your dentist for a checkup every 6 months. The dentist will check your teeth and clean them. This will help keep your gums healthy. You can ask your dentist to show you how to massage your gums.

What else should I know?

Gingivitis can lead to gum disease. Healthy eating helps your gums stay healthy. (See page 46). Cleaning your teeth and massaging your gums will also keep your gums healthy. Some illnesses can cause gum problems. Your dentist may send you to the doctor if your gums do not get healthy.

Gum Disease

What is it?

Gum disease is when gums get infected. This can affect the bones that hold your teeth in place.

What do I see?

Your gums may look red and puffy. They may hurt and bleed easily. You may have bad breath.

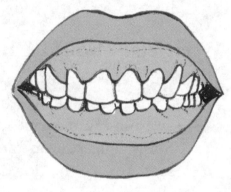

You may not see or feel gum disease until your gums and bone are damaged.

What can I do at home?

- Stop gum disease before it starts.
- Brush your teeth with a soft toothbrush twice a day, and floss your teeth every day.
- Stop smoking.

When should I call the dentist?

Call the dentist if:

- you think you may have gum disease. The dentist can treat it.
- a tooth feels loose (an adult tooth).
- you notice a space between your tooth and gums.
- you have pain, puffiness, or bleeding from your gums.

Gum Disease

See your dentist every 6 months for a checkup. The dentist will check for gum disease and clean your teeth. This will help keep your gums healthy.

What else should I know?

Gum disease is more serious than gingivitis. If you have gum disease, the treatments are more involved. You may have to take antibiotics, have part of your gums cut out, or have a tooth taken out.

The dentist will measure the space between your teeth and gums. There is a small pocket (space) between your tooth and gum at the gum line.

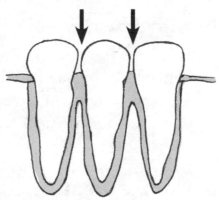

If your gums are healthy, the pocket is not deep. A deep pocket holds more germs and is harder to clean. This can cause gum disease.

You may lose your teeth if you don't take care of gum disease. Teeth can become so loose that you cannot use them to chew. They may fall out, or your dentist may have to take them out.

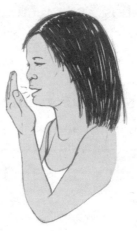

Gum disease may cause bad breath.

Dental Plaque

What is it?

Dental plaque (plak) is a soft, sticky layer of germs on your gums and teeth. It's made of germs, spit, and sugars and starches from food. It always forms and grows in your mouth.

What do I see?

It is hard to see dental plaque. It may be the same color as your teeth. It may feel fuzzy. There is a test you can do to see how much you have. The dentist can give you a pill that you chew up. It turns the plaque pink or purple so you can see it.

What can I do at home?

- Brush your teeth with a soft toothbrush twice a day, and floss your teeth every day. Brushing and flossing is the best way to get rid of plaque.
- Don't eat too much food with lots of sugar.

When should I call the dentist?

See your dentist every 6 months for a checkup. Ask your dentist to show you how to brush and floss your teeth the right way to get rid of plaque.

Dental Plaque

What else should I know?

Dental plaque causes cavities, gingivitis and gum disease. It can also cause you to have bad breath.

Mouthwash alone cannot get rid of dental plaque.

If plaque stays on your teeth, it can harden and become **tartar**. (See next page.)

Dental Tartar

What is it?

Dental tartar is the hard stuff that forms on your teeth. It's made of minerals from spit. Dental plaque can harden into dental tartar.

What do I see?

You may see hard, brittle, crusty stuff on your teeth. You can often see it at the gum line behind your bottom front teeth. You may not see it. It can form below the gum line.

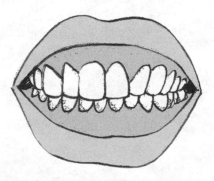

What can I do at home?

- Take good care of your teeth. Brush your teeth with a soft toothbrush twice a day, and floss every day. This will prevent tartar from building up.

- Use "tartar control" toothpaste or mouthwash if your dentist tells you to.

- See your dentist for regular checkups. You can't remove tartar by brushing, but the dentist can get it off.

When should I call the dentist?

See your dentist every 6 months for a checkup. They will remove the tartar as they clean your teeth.

What else should I know?

Germs live and grow in tartar. Tartar under your gum line can give you gum disease.

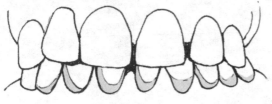

Before

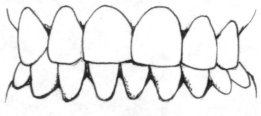

After

27

Dental Care and Cleaning

4

Notes

_____

_____

_____

_____

_____

_____

_____

_____

_____

_____

_____

_____

_____

_____

_____

Toothbrush and Brushing

What is it?

A **toothbrush** is a small brush with a long handle. You use it to clean your teeth. It also gets rid of germs in your mouth.

Did you know?

The bristles on a toothbrush can be soft, medium, or hard. The best kinds are soft. It will say "soft" on the box or brush. Medium and hard bristles can hurt your teeth and gums.

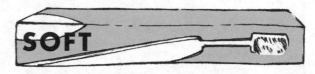

How do I use a toothbrush?

- Hold the handle. Wet the bristles and put some toothpaste on them. You should use toothpaste that has fluoride because it helps keep your teeth strong. Children 2 to 3 years old should only have a small smear on the brush. Those older than 3 and adults should only use a pea-sized amount of toothpaste. Be gentle when you brush your teeth and gums.

Toothbrush and Brushing

- Brush all 3 sides of your teeth:
    1. The **cheek side** (closest to your cheek and lips)
    2. The **tongue side** (closest to your tongue)
    3. The **chewing side** (the side that mashes your food)

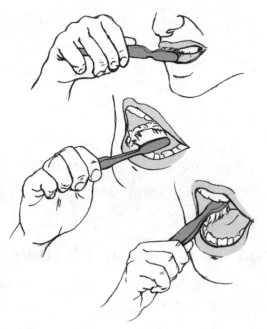

<u>When you brush the cheek side and the tongue side:</u> Brush the sides of your teeth and your gum line gently. Move the toothbrush in small circles. Make sure to brush behind your front teeth. Turn the toothbrush in different directions to reach each tooth.

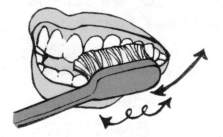

<u>When you brush the chewing side:</u> Put the toothbrush against where your teeth do the biting. Brush back and forth.

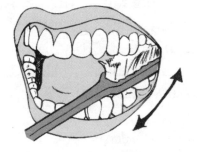

Toothbrush and Brushing

- Brush your teeth for 2 minutes 2 times a day. Test yourself. Use a clock to see how long you brush. You could brush while you listen to a whole song on the radio.

- After you brush your teeth, spit out the toothpaste. Rinse your mouth with water and spit again. Rinse off your toothbrush and stand it up so it can dry.

- Brush your teeth when you wake up in the morning and before you go to bed at night.

What else should I know?

Children and adults use different size toothbrushes. Children have smaller mouths and teeth.

Some toothbrushes use batteries. They are called electric toothbrushes. The power makes the bristles turn and helps you brush. Electric toothbrushes are good if you have trouble using a regular toothbrush. Ask your dentist what kind of toothbrush is best for you.

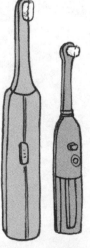

Do not share your toothbrush with anyone, not even a family member. You can spread germs if you share your toothbrush. Get a new toothbrush after you are sick. That way you won't get sick again from the germs on your toothbrush.

Toothbrush and Brushing

When you are done brushing your teeth, store your toothbrush with the brush up, so it can dry. Don't let it touch another toothbrush.

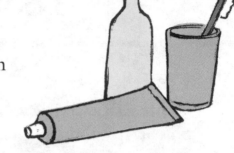

Adults should get a new toothbrush every 3 months. Get a new one sooner if the bristles start to lose their shape. They can lose their shape fast if you don't brush the right way. Children need a new toothbrush more often than adults. They wear out their toothbrushes faster. Get a new brush for your child when the bristles look worn, or every 2 months, whichever comes first.

You need to get all the food out of your teeth before you go to sleep at night. Don't snack after you brush your teeth at night.

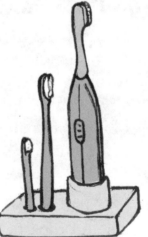

Toothpaste

What is it?

Toothpaste is what you put on your toothbrush to help clean your teeth. It comes in a tube or pump. It takes away stains and gets rid of germs. Toothpaste with fluoride also helps prevent cavities. **Cavities** are holes in your teeth. (See page 18.)

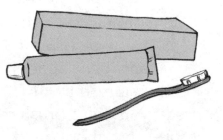

How do I use toothpaste?

- Squeeze the tube. Put a small amount of toothpaste on the bristles of your toothbrush. Use an amount that is the size of a pea. For children 2 to 3 years old, use a smaller amount just a smear.

- Brush correctly. (See page 31).

- The toothpaste should make **foam** (small bubbles or suds). The foam should cover all of your teeth.

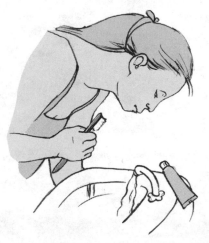

34

Toothpaste

- Spit out the toothpaste when you are done brushing. Rinse your mouth with water to get all the toothpaste out. Don't swallow it.

- Rinse your toothbrush.

What else should I know?

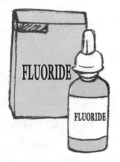

Most toothpaste has a mineral in it called **fluoride**. It makes your teeth stronger and prevents cavities. Read more about fluoride on page 52.

Adults and older kids should use toothpaste that has fluoride in it. But you must be able to spit it out. Fluoride is not good if you swallow it. Children who are not old enough to spit should not use toothpaste with fluoride.

Use toothpaste that is accepted by the American Dental Association. It will have those words or "ADA Accepted" on the box.

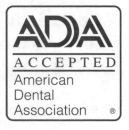

Floss

What is it?

Floss is a special string used to clean between your teeth. It is also called **dental floss**. It is used to clean the sides of a tooth that are next to the tooth in front or behind it. A tooth has 5 sides. The chewing (top) side, the cheek side, and the tongue side. The other two sides are the ones that touch the tooth in front and the tooth behind.

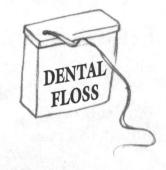

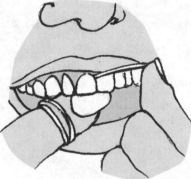

Did you know?

Floss cleans places where your toothbrush can't reach. It cleans between your teeth and under your gums. It helps get rid of food between your teeth. It helps get rid of the germs that cause cavities and gum disease.

Floss comes in different types. All types of floss are OK to use.

- **Dental tape** is wide like small tape. Wide floss is good if you have large gaps between your teeth.
- Some floss is like thin string for smaller spaces.

- **Waxed floss** has wax on it. This makes it slide easier into the small spaces between teeth.

- Some floss tastes like mint.

How do I use floss?

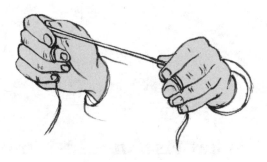

- Pull about 18 inches of floss from the box. This is about the length from your fingertips to your elbow. The box should have a sharp edge to cut the floss after you pull some out.

- Wrap the floss gently and lightly around your middle finger on each hand.

- Put your hands about 1 inch apart. Hold the floss between them in a straight line.

- Use your index finger to slide the floss gently between your teeth. Wiggle the floss back and forth until it gently touches your gum.

- Floss gently and not too deep. Never push the floss too hard. You can cut your gums.

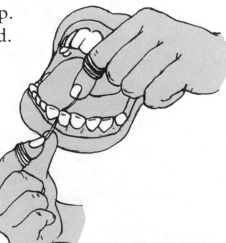

- Slide the floss in a C shape as you follow the shape of your tooth. Move the floss up and down. Do not rub the floss from side to side like you are shining shoes.

- Follow the line of the tooth. Move the floss to the point just under your gum line. Floss slowly and gently.

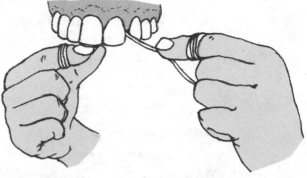

- Be sure to floss behind the last tooth on each side.

- Ask your dentist how to floss the right way.

What else should I know?

Flossing is just as important as brushing your teeth. You should floss once a day. It should take 2 or 3 minutes. Do not hurry.

Flossing may make your gums bleed a bit at first. The gums will stop bleeding and heal. If your gums don't stop bleeding or they hurt a lot, call your dentist.

Flossing may be hard for you to do. Don't give up. It may take 2 weeks to learn to floss well. If it is too hard to use your fingers, try a **floss holder**. This is a tool that holds the floss for you. Some people find this easier to use.

Mouthwash (Mouth Rinse)

What is it?

Mouthwash is a liquid. You swish it around in your mouth and spit it out. It helps to wash germs away and make your mouth healthier. It may also make your breath smell better for a little while.

How do I use mouthwash?

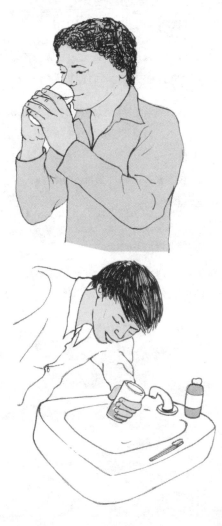

- Pour a small amount of mouthwash into a cup, then pour it into your mouth.

- Swish it around in your mouth for about 30 seconds, then spit it out.

- You can use mouthwash before or after you floss and brush. If you like you can rinse with plain water after you floss and brush.

Mouthwash (Mouth Rinse)

What else should I know?

Never swallow mouthwash. Only use it if you know how to spit out. Mouthwash can make children sick if they swallow it. If you think a child has swallowed some, call the local poison control center right away: (800) 222-1222. Tell them how much was swallowed. They will tell you what to do.

Mouthwash comes in different flavors. Most kinds have alcohol in them to kill the germs in your mouth. Some have no alcohol. The label says "alcohol-free."

Mouthwash can help clean your mouth if you wear braces (wires that make your teeth straight).

Mouthwash alone cannot clean your teeth. You need to brush your teeth with a soft toothbrush twice a day and floss once a day. Mouthwash can be used before or after you brush and floss.

Ask your dentist if you should use mouthwash.

Tongue Scraper

What is it?

A **tongue scraper** is like a small plastic rake. You use it to clean the top of your tongue.

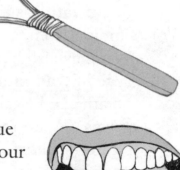

How do I use a tongue scraper?

- Hold the handle and put the tongue scraper all the way to the back of your tongue.
- Gently drag the tongue scraper to the front of your tongue. Rinse it off.
- Do it again, like you are raking leaves in your yard.

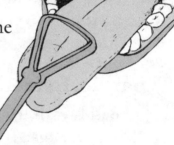

What else should I know?

Go far back on the top of your tongue, but not so far that it's uncomfortable. Do not scrape too hard or make your tongue bleed. Be gentle.

After 2 weeks you should be used to the tongue scraper. It takes germs off your tongue and helps stop bad breath.

Some people brush their tongues with a toothbrush. This is OK.

Bad Breath

What is it?

Bad breath is a bad smell coming from your mouth. You may also have a bad taste in your mouth. Bad breath can be caused by germs in your mouth, cigarette smoking, a cavity, an infection in your mouth, or a problem somewhere else in your body.

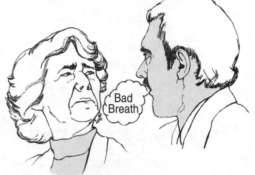

Bad Breath

What do I smell?

Bad breath may smell like rotten eggs. You will not always know you have it because we can't always smell our own breath. Someone else may have to tell you.

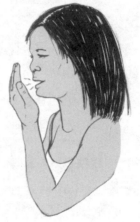

What can I do at home?

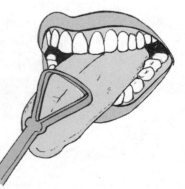

- Brush your teeth with a soft toothbrush twice a day and floss once a day. (Floss is cleaning between your teeth. (See page 37 to learn how to floss.)

- Do not smoke because smoking can cause bad breath.

- Foods like onions, garlic, coffee, and some spicy foods may cause bad breath.

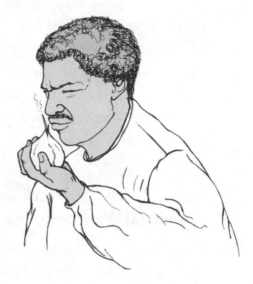

When should I call the dentist?

Call the dentist if you think you are having a problem with bad breath. The dentist will check to see if it is coming from a tooth infection or gum disease. The dentist may have you see a doctor if he or she thinks the bad breath is not coming from your mouth.

What else should I know?

If you do not floss and brush well, food can stay in your mouth, collect germs, and cause bad breath. Food that is stuck in your mouth can rot and cause bad breath. Food can be stuck in between your teeth or under your gums. Mouthwashes will not get rid of bad breath. They will only hide it for about 15 minutes. If you have dentures, food stuck on the dentures can give you bad breath.

Most of the time the cause of bad breath is in your mouth. Sometimes, however, it is caused by something in the lungs, stomach, or another part of the body. Some other causes of bad breath can be, medicines you are taking, or diabetes or blood sugar that is not in good control.

Bad Breath

Spit (saliva) washes off some of the germs in our mouth. You make more saliva when you are awake than when you are asleep. So when you are sleeping, your mouth can get dry. And because you swallow less while sleeping, the germs in your mouth can grow. When you wake up in the morning, you can have bad breath.

Most mouthwash does not work for very long. A mouthwash may work longer if it has **chlorine dioxide, essential oils,** or **zinc chloride**.

Children, teens and even grown-ups may sometimes get a little lazy with brushing, flossing. We all should be reminded that these good habits will keep their teeth and mouths healthy. They will also help prevent bad breath.

A Healthy Diet

5

Notes

A Healthy Diet

What is it?

Eating a **healthy diet** means eating foods that keep your body healthy. The same foods that keep your body healthy also keep your teeth healthy.

Did you know?

Eating well helps keep your gums and teeth strong. You should eat foods that don't help **cavities** (holes) get started in your teeth.

A healthy diet has enough **carbohydrates** (kar-boh-**hye**-drates). These are things in food that give you energy.

You should eat the right amount of fat. The type of fat you eat also is important. Healthy fats give you energy. Your body stores them to keep you warm.

Protein (**proh**-teen) helps you build muscles, organs and more.

Healthy foods have **vitamins** and **minerals**. (See page 49.)

Carbohydrates are found in:

- Fruits
- Vegetables
- Grains
- Rice

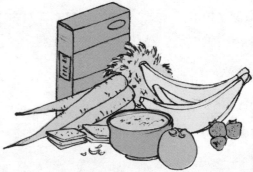

A Healthy Diet

You can find **grains** in breads and cereals. Some grains are:

- Wheat
- Rye
- Oats
- Barley

Healthy fats are in foods like:

- Olive oil
- Nuts
- Fish
- Soybeans
- Peanut butter
- Avocados
- Yogurt
- Olives

Some less healthy fats are the ones that come from animals, like butter, lard and fatty meats.

Protein comes from foods like:

- Meat
- Eggs
- Fish
- Chicken
- Beans
- Tofu

Milk has carbohydrates, fat, and protein.

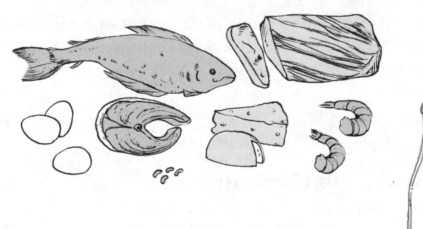

A Healthy Diet

What can I do at home?

- Eat a balanced diet. That means you eat some carbohydrates, some fat, and some protein.

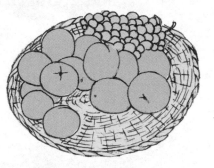

- Try to eat the healthy fats and less of the unhealthy fats.

- Eat lots of fruits and vegetables.

- Eat dark bread, pastas, and cereals for grain. (Dark grains are healthier than white ones. For example, whole wheat bread and brown rice are better than white bread and white rice.)

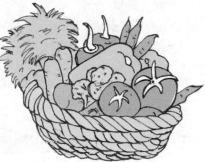

- Do not eat a lot of sugar or sugary foods. Candy, cake, sodas, and cookies have a lot of sugar. If you do eat cake, cookies, or candy, eat them at meal time. Swish and swallow with water to clear them out of your mouth afterwards. Don't snack too much between meals. Stay away from hard candy because it lasts a long time in your mouth.

- Brush and floss your teeth after you eat sweets or at least rinse your mouth out with water.

When should I call the dentist?

See the dentist every 6 months for a checkup. Ask the dentist about your diet if you want advice.

48

Vitamins and Minerals

What are they?

Vitamins and **minerals** are good things found in food.
They help keep your teeth and gums strong and healthy.
They also keep the rest of your body healthy!

What do I see?

Fruits, vegetables, milk and
other healthy foods have
vitamins and minerals. Some
examples are vitamin A, vitamin
C, calcium, and folic acid.

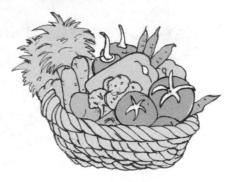

What can I do at home?

- Eat foods with a lot of
  vitamins and minerals.
  The best foods are fruits,
  vegetables, whole grains
  and low-fat milk.

- Learn about the vitamins
  and minerals in food.
  You want to know which
  ones are good for you
  and your teeth. (See the
  chart on page 51.)

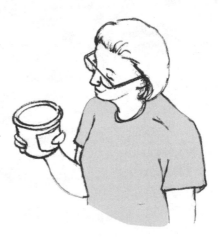

Vitamins and Minerals

- Read the labels on the food you eat. Labels show what kinds of vitamins and minerals the food has.

- Take vitamin pills if your doctor or dentist tells you to. Ask which ones to take so you get enough vitamins and minerals. Vitamin pills don't take the place of food. You take them with food.

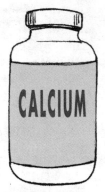

What else should I know?

Good food helps make your whole body healthy: your hair, skin, eyes, heart, bones, and teeth.

Fruits and vegetables are good snacks. Both have lots of vitamins and minerals. Most candy has no vitamins or minerals.

Vitamins and Minerals

Vitamin	What Does it Do?	Where do I get it?
Vitamin A	• Protects mouth • Forms teeth • Forms bones • Helps you see in the dark	Egg yolks, milk, Sweet potatoes, Carrots, Pumpkins, Cantaloupes, Apricots, Cheddar Cheese, Liver, Broccoli
Vitamin B-12	• Prevents cracks and sores in the mouth and lips • Prevents bone loss	Beef, Pork, Fish, Eggs, Dairy products
Vitamin B-6	• Prevents canker sores • Prevents bad breath	Fortified cereals, Meats, Cabbage, Potatoes, Beans, Fish, Milk
Folic Acid	• Taken during pregnancy to prevent birth defects	Whole-wheat foods, Green vegetables
Vitamin C	• Healthy for teeth, bones and gums • Helps put iron into body • Prevents gums from bleeding • Helps body heal wounds	Oranges, Strawberries, Cantaloupe, Red peppers, Papayas, Potatoes
Vitamin D	• Forms teeth and bones • Prevents cavities • Helps put calcium into teeth • Without this vitamin, bones would be soft	Sunlight, Milk, Eggs, Sardines, Salmon, Fortified breakfast cereals
Vitamin K	• Helps the blood to clot (thicken and stop bleeding) • Prevents the gums from bleeding	Spinach, Broccoli, Brussels sprouts, Strawberries, Milk, Eggs, Corn
Calcium	• Helps form bones and teeth • Very important to have during child's early years and teenage years	Milk, Cheese, Yogurt, Broccoli, Dark leafy vegetables like spinach
Phosphorus	• Helps form bones and teeth	Dairy products, Meat, Fish, Chicken

Fluoride

What is it?

Fluoride (floor-ide) is a mineral. It makes teeth stronger and helps stop cavities.

What do I see?

While you don't see fluoride, there are several ways for you to get the fluoride you need:

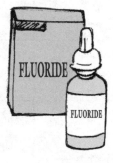

- Fluoride may be in the water from your tap.

- Fluoride is in some toothpastes and mouth rinses. Ask your dentist if your child needs a mouth rinse with fluoride.

- Dentists can give you fluoride pills or drops. Ask the dentist if your child needs them. The dentist can prescribe (order) this kind of fluoride so your child gets the right amount.

- Dentists and hygienists can also put fluoride on your teeth.

- Very small amounts of fluoride are in most foods and drinks.

Fluoride

What can I do at home?

- Find out if your town puts fluoride in the tap water. If it does, then drink that instead of bottled water. Most bottled water does not contain fluoride and so you may be missing the decay-stopping effect of fluoride in tap water.

- Use toothpaste or mouthwash with fluoride in it. This is for adults and older children who know how to spit out. Children under three should use only a smear, Children ages 3 to 6 should only use a pea-sized amount.

Fluoride?

When should I call the dentist?

Ask your dentist if there is fluoride in the drinking water where you live.

What else should I know?

Ask your dentist if you are getting the right amount of fluoride.

The right amount of fluoride makes your teeth stronger.

Stronger teeth fight cavities better.

Fluoride

Toothpaste with fluoride should have the ADA (American Dental Association) Seal of Acceptance on the box.

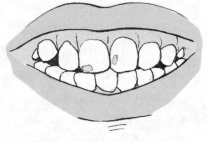

Children under 3 years old should only use a smear of toothpaste with fluoride in it. Child under between 3 and 6 years old should only use a pea-sized amount. Too much fluoride can give growing teeth brown or white spots.

The amount of fluoride in drinking water is very small. It is okay to swallow and helps your teeth. The amount in toothpaste is good for brushing your teeth, but it is too much to swallow.

Pregnancy

6

Notes

55

Pregnancy

What is it?

Pregnancy is when a baby is growing inside a woman. The baby grows inside for about 40 weeks.

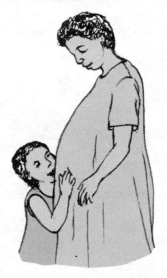

What do I see?

Your body changes in many ways. Your tummy gets big and round as the baby grows. You gain weight. You may also see changes in your gums.

What can I do at home?

- Take care of yourself.
- Eat foods that are good for you. (See pages 46–51.)
- See a doctor to find out if you are going to have a baby. Make regular doctor visits the whole time you are pregnant.
- Do what the doctor says about food, vitamins, exercise, sleep, and taking care of yourself.
- Take care of your mouth and teeth.

When should I call the dentist?

Tell your dentist as soon as you know you are pregnant.

What else should I know?

See your dentist for regular cleanings during your pregnancy. Keeping your mouth healthy will help your baby be healthy.

Your baby's teeth are forming as the baby grows inside you. These teeth start to form in your second month of pregnancy.

Sometimes pregnant women get **gingivitis** (**jin**-ji-vi-tis). This is a problem with your gums. (See page 20.) You can avoid it by brushing with a soft toothbrush 2 times a day and flossing once a day. Learn more about gum problems on page 22.

Read the book "What to Do When You're Having a Baby." You can buy this book from IHA. Look at the back cover of this book to find a phone number and website. You can order the book by phone or online.

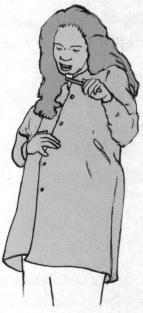

Eating Right
During Pregnancy

What is it?

It's eating good food to help your baby grow the right way. The food you eat also goes to your baby.

What can I do at home?

- Do not drink wine, beer, or any alcohol while you are pregnant.

- Do not smoke while you are pregnant. Stop smoking when you first plan on having a baby.

- Stop taking any street drugs before you get pregnant and all through your pregnancy.

- Eat foods that have the nutrients (noo-tree-uhnts) you need. (See page 46.)

To get vitamins and minerals: Eat lots of fruits and vegetables, whole grains, and dairy products like milk, eggs and yogurt.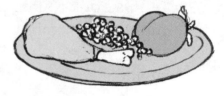

To get protein: Eat chicken, fish and other lean meats, eggs, beans, tofu and milk.

To get carbohydrates: Eat whole grain breads, pasta, rice, cereals and other whole grains

- Eat foods with lots of calcium (**kal**-see-uhm). It makes your baby's teeth and bones stronger.
  - Dairy products like milk, yogurt and cheese

- Green leafy vegetables like collard greens, mustard greens and spinach
- Tofu, kidney beans and soybeans

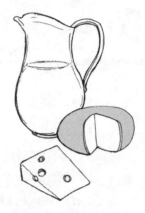

If you don't eat dairy products, ask your doctor how to get enough calcium for you and your baby.

- Ask your doctor if the medicines you take are safe for you and your growing baby.

- Take vitamin pills with **folic acid**. Your doctor will order these for you when you want to get pregnant. You will take these until after the first 3 months of pregnancy.

When should I call the dentist?

Call the dentist if:

- your teeth hurt when you eat or drink.
- your teeth hurt when you have hot or cold food or drinks.
- your gums hurt or bleed when touched.

See the dentist every 6 months for a checkup.

What else should I know?

Drinking alcohol or smoking can hurt your baby as it is growing inside you. Don't drink or smoke when you are pregnant.

Many drugs can hurt your baby as it grows inside you. Stop taking all drugs. Ask the doctor if you feel you need to take medicine.

Your Gums During Pregnancy

What is it?

Gums are the pink part around
your teeth. When you are
pregnant, germs in your mouth
can make your gums hurt. This is
called **gingivitis**. (See page 19 to
learn more about gingivitis.)

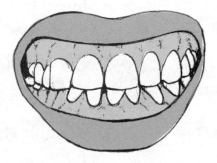

What do I see?

When you have gingivitis, your gums get more red, and
may hurt. They may also look puffy, or they may bleed.

What can I do at home?

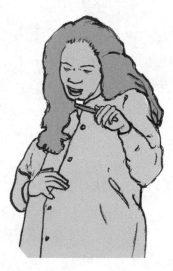

- Brush your teeth with a soft
  toothbrush twice a day and
  floss once a day. This will help
  get rid of the germs.

- See your dentist for cleanings
  every 6 months even when you
  are pregnant.

When should I call the dentist?

Call the dentist if:

- your gums hurt or bleed.

Your Gums During Pregnancy

Keep up with your 6-month checkups. Be sure to see the dentist at least one time when you are pregnant. This is to make sure you don't have cavities, gum disease, or an infection. Make sure to tell the dentist you are pregnant.

What else should I know?

Keep your mouth healthy. This helps keep your baby healthy.

Your body makes hormones when you are pregnant. These help your baby grow, but they can make the germs in your mouth hurt your gums more. The germs from your mouth can go to your blood and then to the baby. This can sometimes make the baby be born too early and too small. If you get rid of the germs, they won't go to the baby.

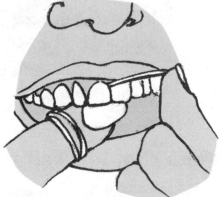

If you have trouble with your gums when you are pregnant, you need to get treated by your dentist. These problems could go on even while you are nursing your baby. Your gums may need extra care for 3-6 months after your baby is born.

Your gums may hurt and bleed a little when you first floss. Do not stop flossing. After about 2 weeks this should stop.

Your gums should not hurt and bleed when you brush and floss at home.

Cavities During Pregnancy

What is it?

A **cavity** is a hole in your tooth. It is caused by germs in your mouth.

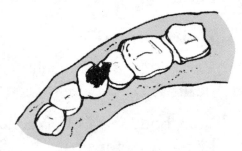

What do I see?

Most of the time you can't see the hole. The dentist must look for it.

What can I do at home?

- Brush your teeth at least twice a day and floss at least once a day.
- Use a tongue scraper or toothbrush to clean your tongue. It helps get rid of germs.
- Try not to eat and drink things that have a lot of sugar.
- Do not take drugs or medicines unless your doctor tells you to.

When should I call the dentist?

Call the dentist if:

- you see a hole in your tooth.
- your tooth hurts, even if you don't see a hole.

Cavities During Pregnancy

Keep up with your 6-month checkups. Be sure to see the dentist at least one time when you are pregnant. This is to make sure you don't have cavities, gum disease, or an infection. Make sure to tell your dentist you are pregnant.

What else should I know?

If your mouth is clean and healthy, your baby will be healthier.

It is safe to see a dentist while you are pregnant. Pregnant women who go to the dentist every 6 months have fewer cavities.

You might **vomit** (throw up) when you are pregnant during the first 3 months. Vomit on your teeth can cause cavities. Rinse out your mouth after throwing up. Use a half a teaspoon of baking soda stirred into a glass of water. Then spit it out. Do not drink it. Do not brush or floss your teeth right after you throw up or right after you rinse them.

Toothache During Pregnancy

What is it?

A toothache is pain in your mouth or in your teeth. Your tooth may hurt when you eat or drink hot or cold things. It may hurt when you bite.

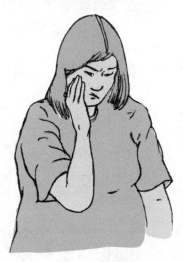

What do I see?

You may not see anything at all. Your gums might look puffy or red.

What can I do at home?

- Eat the right foods and take care of your teeth so you don't get cavities.
- If you get a cavity or have a toothache, don't try to fix it at home. Call your dentist.

When should I call the dentist?

Call your dentist if:

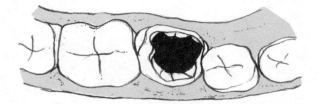

- your tooth hurts.
- you see a hole in your tooth.

What else should I know?

Your dentist should talk to your doctor before you take any medicine for your teeth. Some medicines are not good to take when you are pregnant. For example, if you take tetracycline, it can make dark marks on your baby's teeth.

Your Child's Teeth (Birth to Age Five)

7

Notes

_____

_____

_____

_____

_____

_____

_____

_____

_____

_____

_____

_____

_____

Caring for Your Baby's Teeth

What is it?

Caring for your baby's teeth is making sure their teeth and mouth are healthy. You do this by cleaning and checking them.

What do I see?

At first you can't see your baby's teeth. They are forming inside the baby's gums. Teeth may start to pop out from the gums when the baby is about 6 months old. Some come earlier or later. This is OK. These first teeth are called **baby teeth** or **primary teeth**. Your child's baby teeth should all be the same color.

A child will have all 20 baby teeth by about age 3. **Adult teeth** are forming under their gums. These are also called **permanent teeth**.

What can I do at home?

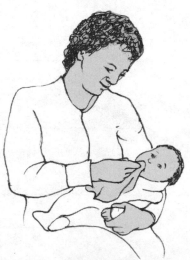

- Start cleaning your baby's mouth when baby is a few days old. Use a clean, damp washcloth wrapped around your finger. Gently wipe baby's gums after feeding your baby. This helps baby get used to dental care at an early age.

Caring for Your Baby's Teeth

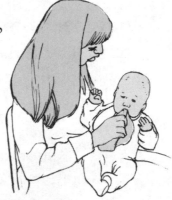

- When your baby gets teeth, use a wet, soft, child-size toothbrush to clean them. You can also use a clean, damp, soft washcloth. Do this in the morning and at night, before bed. Use a tiny smear of toothpaste.

- Learn what your baby's teeth and mouth look like. That way you can tell if something changes. You will know if there may be a problem.

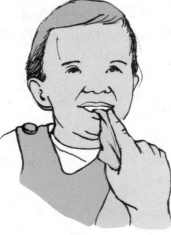

- Help your child brush using a soft toothbrush and floss until he or she can do these things well on their own. Your child can start using toothpaste when they are three and are able to spit it out when brushing is done.

When should I call the dentist or doctor?

Call the dentist if:

- your baby's teeth have white, yellow, or brown spots.
- your baby has sores in the mouth.

You should make your baby's first dental checkup by the time he or she is 1 year old. Children should see the dentist every 6 months. The dentist will clean their teeth and check for cavities and gum problems. The dentist will also teach you what to expect as your baby grows.

What else should I know?

Babies use their teeth to eat, talk and smile. Baby teeth are important because they save space for adult teeth.

Germs that cause cavities live in your baby's mouth even before teeth come in. Germs go from your mouth to the baby's mouth when the baby puts its fingers in your mouth. Kissing baby on the lips can also pass germs. Sharing food with your baby or tasting your baby's food to see if it is too hot can also spread germs. As babies explore, they often put things in their mouths. This is another way that germs can spread.

Parents should keep their own mouths clean and healthy. Do this by brushing twice a day and flossing once a day.

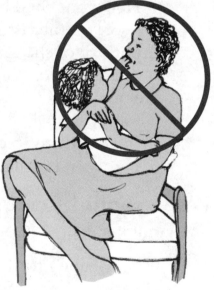

Bottle Rot
(Early Childhood Cavities)

What is it?

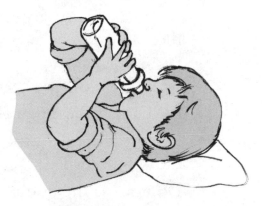

Bottle rot is when the baby's front top teeth rot. This happens when sweet liquids from a bottle sit in the baby's mouth. Sweet liquids include formula, milk, and juice. Bottle rot most often happens when babies get a bottle at naptime or bedtime. It can also occur in babies who are breastfed.

What do I see?

The top 4 front teeth may have white, yellow, or brown spots. You may also see sores in your baby's mouth.

You baby may be in pain and have trouble chewing. Your baby may stop eating because their mouth hurts.

What can I do at home?

- Teach your baby good habits. Don't start bad habits. It is easier to learn good habits than to change bad ones.
- Sing, read, or rock your baby without a bottle to help them calm down or get to sleep.

Bottle Rot (Early Childhood Cavities)

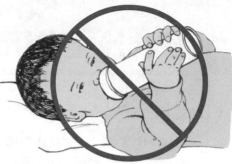

- Do not put your baby to bed with a bottle. This includes naptime and bedtime. Milk, juice, and formula all have sugar in them.

- Do not use the bottle to stop your baby from being fussy or bored. This can give the baby bad eating habits.

- Do not give the bottle as a reward, or take it away when the child is bad.

- Do not use the bottle or breast as a pacifier.

- Hold your baby while feeding. Don't lay your baby down with a bottle.

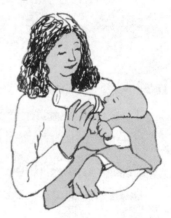

- If you breastfeed, stop when your baby falls asleep. You want the baby to swallow all the milk in their mouth. That way the milk doesn't stay on the teeth when baby sleeps.

- Teach your child to drink only water at night. If your child is used to drinking juice or something else when going to sleep, try this plan: Each night mix more and more water into the bottle. Try one third water the first night, half the second night, and all water the third.

Bottle Rot (Early Childhood Cavities)

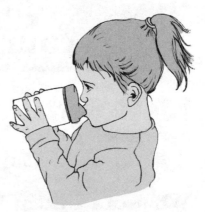

- Start to teach your baby to drink from a sippy cup at 5-12 months old.

- Stop using a bottle when your baby is about 12 months old, or when your baby has teeth.

When should I call the dentist?

Call the dentist if:

- you see white, yellow, or brown spots on your baby's top front teeth. This may mean your baby has bottle rot.

What else should I know?

Bottle rot can cause many problems for your baby. It can:

- hurt how well your baby grows.
- cause sickness (infection).
- hurt your baby's adult teeth when they come in.
- make your baby's teeth crooked. This can cause speech problems.

If your baby gets bottle rot, the dentist will need to take care of your baby's teeth. It may be hard for the baby to sit still for the dentist. The dentist may need to use medicine to calm or put your baby to sleep in order to work on their teeth. Talk to your dentist about what's best for you and your child.

Fluoride and Your Baby's Teeth

What is it?

Fluoride is a mineral that protects your teeth so they don't get cavities.

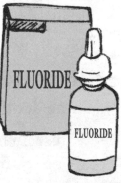

What can I do at home?

• Drink water with fluoride in it. Find out if the water that comes from your tap has fluoride. Some water you buy at the store will have fluoride. This will be on the label.

When should I call the dentist?

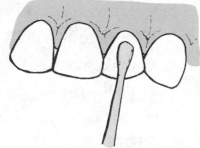

Ask your dentist if your child gets enough fluoride. Ask if there is fluoride in your drinking water. The dentist may order fluoride drops if your baby is more than 6 months old. They may also put fluoride on your child's teeth with a brush.

Fluoride and Your Baby's Teeth

What else should I know?

Some towns put fluoride in the tap water to help people have healthy teeth. (You can't see it.) Ask your dentist if your town's water has fluoride. If it doesn't, your dentist can order fluoride pills or drops. If you get 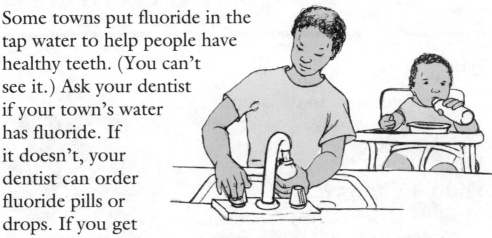 fluoride drops for your child, follow the directions. Make sure to use them right.

It is important to get the right amount of fluoride. Ask your dentist or pediatrician about your baby's fluoride needs.

A Visit to the Dentist

What is it?

Regular visits to the dentist are important to keep your child's teeth healthy.

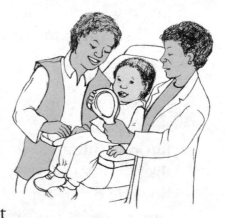

Did you know?

The dentist will look for cavities and fix any problems with your baby's teeth or gums. The dentist will also teach you how to take care of your child's teeth.

The dentist will:

- tell you how to feed your baby so baby has healthy teeth.
- teach you how to take care of your baby's teeth to stop cavities before they start.
- make sure your baby gets the right amount of fluoride.
- tell you how to stop accidents that can hurt your baby's teeth.

What do I see?

The dentist might ask you to hold your baby in a special way so he or she can look in the baby's mouth. You will put your baby in your lap with its legs around your waist. You and the dentist sit facing each other with your knees touching. Your baby lies across both your lap and the dentist's. The dentist likely will show your child a toothbrush.

A Visit to the Dentist

What can I do at home?

- Ask your baby's doctor for the name of a children's dentist. You can also talk with family and friends for a children's dentist.

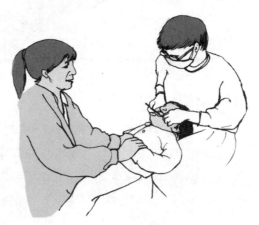

- Take your baby to the dentist by the time they are one year old.

When should I call the dentist?

You should call the dentist if something happens to one of your baby's teeth. If a tooth is cracked or is knocked out, be sure to call the dentist right away.

What else should I know?

A healthy mouth has gums that are firm and pink, white teeth, and have no mouth sores.

Some dentists work only with children. They are called **pediatric dentists**. They know how to work with children to make the visit more fun.

Babies and children with special needs may need extra care and cleaning of their teeth. Ask your dentist or pediatrician about special ways you can help your child have clean and healthy teeth.

Teething

What is it?

Teething is when a baby's teeth start to come out of the gums for the first time. Babies start teething around 4 months of age. Most children have all their baby teeth by the time they are 3 years old.

What do I see?

The baby's gums may look red or swollen. Baby's gums may be tender. Teething can hurt and make your baby fussy and cranky. Your baby may drool. Babies may put things in their mouth more often when they are teething. Biting and chewing on things makes their mouth feel better.

What can I do at home?

- Gently rub and clean where the teeth are coming in. Use a clean, damp cloth.
- Give the baby something safe to bite. A teething ring is good. But do not give your baby a teething ring with liquid in it.

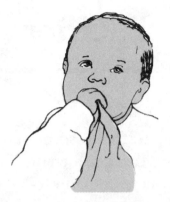

- Let your baby chew on a clean, wet washcloth that has been in the freezer. (Don't keep it in the freezer for more than 30 minutes.)
- Do not rub numbing gels on the baby's gums. Numbing gels make the baby's gums lose feeling but can cause a serious health problem.
- Do not rub liquor (booze) or alcohol on the baby's gums.
- Never cut the baby's gums to help a tooth come out.

When should I call the dentist?

Call the dentist if:

Your baby is still crying or cranky after trying the tips above.

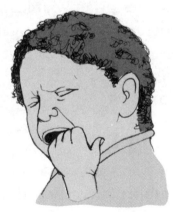

The dentist can tell you if you should give your baby medicine for pain.

What else should I know?

Teething does not cause a fever.

Pacifiers and Thumbs

What is it?

A **pacifier** is something you can get for your baby to suck on for comfort.

Did you know?

Some babies feel better when they have something in their mouth to suck on. Sucking is normal for babies. Many babies suck their thumbs or fingers for comfort. Some babies like to use a pacifier for comfort.

What do I see?

A pacifier is made of rubber. It's shaped like a nipple.

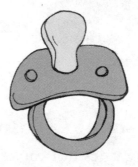

What can I do at home?

- Give your baby a safe, clean pacifier. Make sure it is strong. A pacifier is safe if:
- it's all one piece.

Pacifiers and Thumbs

- it's made of a material that is safe to go in a baby's mouth.

- it has a mouth guard with 2 air holes in it.

- it's big enough so the baby cannot swallow it.

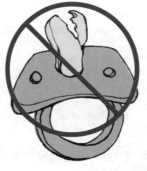

- Check the nipple sometimes by pulling on it. Make sure it isn't loose. It should not come off in the baby's mouth.

- Throw away the pacifier if it is worn out. Get a new one if it is torn or if there are cracks in it.

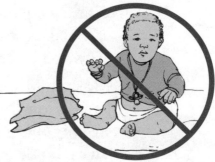

- Never hang a pacifier or anything around a child's neck. It could choke them and cause death.

- Never tie a pacifier to the crib or bed.

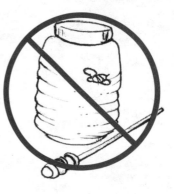

- Never put sweet liquid or honey on a pacifier. This can cause cavities. Children younger than 1 year should **never** eat honey. It can make them sick.

When should I call the dentist?

You should talk to your dentist if your child sucks their thumb or fingers or uses a pacifier. The dentist may check the child's bite. The bite is the way your child's top and bottom teeth come together.

Call the dentist if you are worried about your child sucking a pacifier or thumb. Call your doctor right away if your baby swallows a piece of their pacifier.

What else should I know?

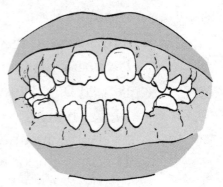

- Using a pacifier for too long can make the child's teeth crowded or crooked.

- Most children stop using a pacifier on their own. Most stop by the time they are 3 or 4 years old.

Tooth Accidents

What is it?

Accidents are when something unplanned happens, like a fall. Someone may get hurt. Sometimes babies and toddlers hurt their mouth, lips, tongue, or teeth. They can do this while playing, climbing, running or any other activity. A child can also bite their lip or mouth while chewing on something else.

What do I see?

Your child may be crying and you may see blood. Blood can come from their gums, tongue, or lips. If they are bleeding, look inside the mouth to see where the blood is coming from.

If your baby has teeth, they may get damaged from a fall or a bad hit in the face. The teeth may get pushed up into the gums, or they may come out of the gums a bit. A piece of the child's tooth may break off. Sometimes whole teeth may come out.

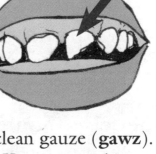

What can I do at home?

- If your child's teeth or gums are bleeding: Put cold water on a clean washcloth or a piece of clean gauze (**gawz**). Gauze is a thin, clean woven cloth. You can use it to wash off blood, or to cover a cut like a bandage. Press the cold gauze or washcloth on the area that is hurt.

- If a tooth is broken: Rinse your child's mouth with warm water. Put a cold washcloth on their face or on the area where the tooth came out. This will help stop swelling.

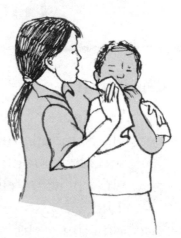

- If the tooth is knocked out completely, put it into a clean container with milk. It's important to keep the tooth moist. (See page 156, "Knocked-out Teeth.")

When should I call the dentist?

Call the dentist if:

- your child hurts their mouth, or hurts their face near their mouth.
- your child gets hurt and has blood on their teeth or gums.
- your child's lip is bitten or bleeding after being hurt.
- your child gets hurt and can't eat cold food without crying.

Keep the emergency phone number of a dentist or dental clinic by your phone. Write it in the front of this book right now.

What else should I know?

If a baby tooth gets hurt, that can hurt the adult tooth under it.

Hand-Foot-Mouth Disease

What is it?

Hand-foot-mouth disease is a sickness caused by a virus. You can get it easily from someone else.

What do I see?

Your child may have a fever of 101 degrees or higher. You may see small bumps in your baby's mouth and on their hands and feet. The bumps look like blisters. You may also see them in the diaper area, or on the legs and arms. Bumps in the mouth can be:

- on the tongue
- on the gums
- inside the lips
- in the cheeks
- near the throat

Your child may not want to eat.

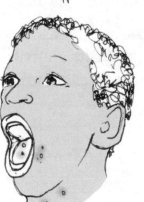

Hand-Foot-Mouth Disease

What can I do at home?

- Call your doctor or dentist before you do anything.
- If your child has a fever, ask your doctor or dentist if you should give your child Tylenol.
- Give your child small amounts of cool water.
- Try to prevent spreading the disease to others:
  - Wash your hands often
  - Do not share food and toys.
  - Have children use their own towels.
  - Keep your child at home.

When should I call the dentist or doctor?

Call the dentist if you see bumps in the baby's mouth. Call your child's doctor if they have a fever to ask whether you should give the child Tylenol.

What else should I know?

The bumps go away after about a week. Hand-foot-mouth disease can spread to other people.

This disease happens more in the summer and the fall.

Hand-foot-mouth disease is different from hoof-and-mouth disease, which affects animals only. People don't get hoof-and-mouth disease, and animals don't get hand-foot-mouth disease.

Your Child's Teeth (Ages Six to Eleven)

8

Notes

_____

_____

_____

_____

_____

_____

_____

_____

_____

_____

_____

_____

_____

_____

_____

The Six-Year Molars

What are they?

The **molars** (**moe**-lurs) are the wide flat teeth in the back of the mouth. They are used to grind and chew food. Most children get these teeth around age 6. They will keep these teeth for the rest of their lives.

What do I see?

At first you may see white tips of the teeth coming out of your child's gums. They come in on the top and bottom.

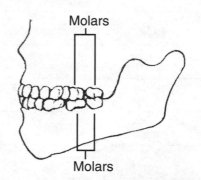

They are in the back of the mouth behind the last baby teeth. (Other adult teeth come in under the baby teeth.)

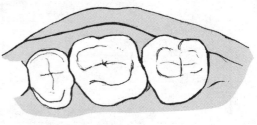

What can I do at home?

• Start to look for the molars when your child is 5 or 6 years old. Look in their mouth about once a week to see if the molars are coming in.

• Take care of the six-year molars. They need extra care when they are starting to come into the mouth. Help your child to keep them clean. Use a small toothbrush to reach back and clean them as soon as they start coming in.

The Six-Year Molars

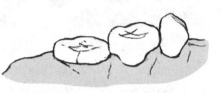

- Use toothpaste with fluoride if your child can spit out. Toothpaste should be the size of a small pea.

- Get your child to brush each morning and each night before bed. And they should floss their teeth one time each day. Help your child brush and floss until they can do it well by themselves.

Did you know?

Most children get their 4 adult six-year molars by first grade. They are the biggest teeth. They are also the widest teeth on the top where they chew and grind food.

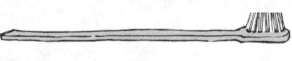

These molars are the most important teeth for a child's bite. The **bite** is the way all the teeth fit together.

Adults use these molars more than other teeth to chew food.

When should I call the dentist?

Call the dentist when you see the adult six-year molars coming in. Your dentist may want to put a plastic coating called a sealant (**see**-luhnt) on the teeth. The dentist may want to do this even while the teeth are still coming in. This will help protect them from cavities.

You can talk to your dentist at your child's 6-month checkup. Your child should see the dentist every 6 months for checkups.

What else should I know?

The six-year molars have the strongest roots. They are important teeth because they help the rest of the teeth line up the way they should. If one of these molars has a cavity or gets knocked out, it will need to be fixed or replaced. Other molars may come in the wrong way if any of the six-year molars are missing.

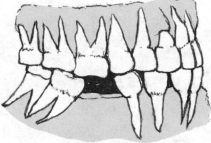

Losing Baby Teeth

What is it?

At some point, children lose their baby teeth and bigger adult teeth come in. These teeth are permanent. When your child is between the ages of 5 and 7, their front teeth will get loose. Then they will fall out. This means the adult teeth are getting ready to come in.

What do I see?

Your child's front baby teeth will feel loose. You can wiggle them back and forth. After some time, they will come out. Sometimes it will bleed a little from the place where the tooth came out.

What can I do at home?

- Reassure your child that losing their baby tooth is normal.

- Let the baby teeth fall out on their own. If you pull out the tooth before it is ready to come out, you will tear the gum and it may bleed. Do not try to pull a tooth out. Do not put a string around the loose tooth and pull.

- Let your child wiggle the tooth, if they want to.

- Give your child soft foods if they have a hard time eating. You can try Jell-O, pudding, yogurt, or cottage cheese.

- Explain what is happening so they are not scared when they have a loose tooth. Some parents give the child a prize when their first tooth comes out.

- If your child's mouth bleeds when a tooth comes out, put clean wet gauze or a wet paper towel in the space where the tooth was. Put light pressure on the towel or gauze and hold it for 3-5 minutes. You can also try putting a warm, wet teabag on the space.

When do I call the dentist or clinic?

Call the dentist if:

- your child is having pain.
- the gum is very puffy and your child has pain.
- if the permanent tooth comes in before the baby tooth come out.
- a back tooth is loose, and your child is having problems biting down.
- there is bleeding for more than 10 minutes after the tooth comes out.

What else should I know?

Your child's gums may be puffy because a new, larger tooth is coming in to replace the baby tooth.

There may also be some bleeding, even when the tooth comes out by itself.

Many children look forward to their first loose tooth.

Losing Baby Teeth Too Early

What is it?

A baby tooth should stay in the mouth until the adult tooth below pushes it out and makes it fall out. Baby teeth can come out early from a cavity or an injury.

What do I see?

If a child loses a baby tooth too early, you will see a space where the tooth was. You will not see an adult tooth coming in. If your child loses a tooth because of cavities, you will see an empty space. The roots of the tooth may still be in the gum.

What can I do at home?

- Look at your child's teeth often. If you see a change, ask your dentist about it.

- Make sure your child brushes twice a day and flosses once a day. This helps prevent cavities. Your child should brush and floss well by the age of 9. You may need to help them before that.

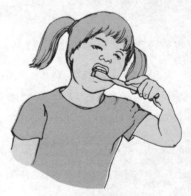

- Make sure your child is getting the right amount of fluoride. Check with your dentist.

- See the dentist for a checkup every 6 months. The dentist will check for cavities.

When do I call the dentist?

Call your dentist right away if a baby tooth comes out too early.

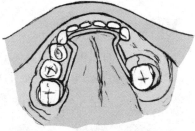

The dentist may need to put in a **space saver**. This helps to keep the space the right size for the adult tooth. Without one, the other teeth can move into the space. They may not leave room for the adult tooth to grow in. The nearby teeth can more into the space in as little as in 6 weeks. The dentist will decide if your child needs a space saver. It will depend on your child's age and which tooth came out. The space saver will usually be kept in until the adult tooth starts to come in. Watch for the adult tooth to start to show if your child has a space saver. Call your dentist when you see it.

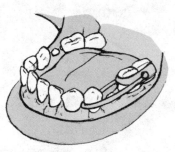

What else should I know?

If a baby tooth comes out too soon and no space saver is put in, the adult tooth may not have room. It could get stuck in the gum.

Some children have a problem saying some letters or words correctly when they are missing one or more baby teeth.

Adult (Permanent) Teeth

What are they?

Adult (permanent) teeth come in when baby teeth are lost. This starts to happen when a child is five or six years old.

What do I see?

Most children lose their bottom 2 front teeth first. Then the adult teeth come in to take their place. Sometimes the adult teeth come in behind the baby teeth before they fall out. It looks like the child has 2 rows of teeth. This is normal.

When the top front adult teeth come in you may see bumps on the edges of them. This is also normal.

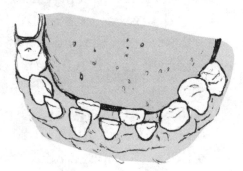

Sometimes you see the six-year molars in the back 4 corners of the mouth first. Each child is different.

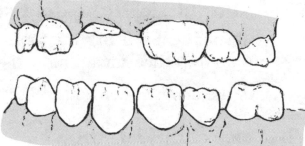

Adult (Permanent) Teeth

What can I do at home?

- Watch for your child's new adult teeth at least once a week. Have your child open their mouth wide so you can see.

- Brush the new teeth well. Use toothpaste with fluoride in it if your child can spit. Use a pea-sized amount.

- Have your child use a small enough toothbrush so that they can reach the teeth in the back of their mouth.

- Some parents find charting the child's success is helpful. You can put stickers on it for prizes when your child remembers to brush 2 times a day and floss every day.

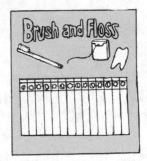

- Check how well your child brushes and flosses their teeth. Brush and floss again if they don't reach each tooth. If it is hard for your child to handle the floss to clean between all of their teeth, a floss fork may help. A floss fork is a plastic floss holder which gives your child a handle to hold. It makes it easier for some people to floss. (See page 38.)

When should I call the dentist?

Call your dentist if an adult tooth comes in on one side, but not on the other side for more than 6 months.

Call the dentist when your child's 6-year molars come in.

What else should I know?

It can take 6 months to a year for an adult tooth to come in.

Adult (Permanent) Teeth

If you see 2 rows of bottom teeth, don't panic. It is OK to have baby teeth and adult teeth at the same time. Use your finger to feel if the baby teeth are loose. The adult teeth (behind the baby teeth) get pushed by the tongue. This can help make the baby teeth get loose and fall out. This should happen in a few weeks.

The dentist will decide if the baby teeth have to be pulled. If this happens, ask your dentist to explain to your child what they will be doing.

Don't worry if you see bumps on the edges of the top front adult teeth. This is normal. The bumps will get smooth from chewing.

Sometimes adult teeth come in with yellow, brown, or white spots on them. There are different things that can cause spots on the adult teeth:

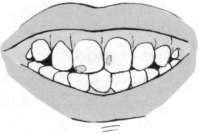

- A tooth can get spots when it is growing in the gum and the child gets a high fever or hurts a baby tooth.

- Too much fluoride during the time teeth are forming under the gums can cause white spots on your child's adult teeth. Ask your dentist about your child's fluoride needs. If you don't brush and floss well, you may get spots from **plaque**. (See page 24.)

Most children lose all their baby teeth by the time they're 12 years old. They will have 28 adult teeth that grow back in. As kids get older their second molars will grow in as well. Then they will have 32 adult teeth.

Sealants

What is it?

A **sealant** is a safe coating that can protect your back teeth. The dentist puts the sealant on top of your back teeth (molars). This keeps out food and germs that make cavities.

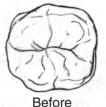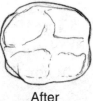

Before   After

What do I see?

The teeth in back called molars have deep grooves. They look like hills and valleys. Sealant on these teeth looks like white or clear paint, but it is not paint.

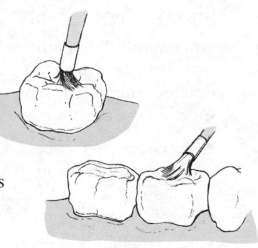

What can I do at home?

• Watch for your child's six-year molars to come in.
• Call your dentist when you see them.

When should I call the dentist?

Call the dentist when you see the tops of your child's molars coming in. The dentist will decide when it's time to put on the sealant. Usually molars get sealant. The dentist may also want to seal some baby teeth.

What else should I know?

Most cavities in children over 5 years old are on the **chewing surface** of the tooth. This is the top part of the molars. (See the pictures on page 98.)

Sealants are safe and easy for the dentist to put on each tooth. Sealed molars are less likely to get cavities. This can save money because sealants cost much less than a filling.

Bad Bite

What is it?

A **bad bite** means the teeth, lips, and jaw do not line up the way they should.

What do I see?

Your child's teeth may look crooked. The top teeth may stick out too far over the bottom teeth. Or when the teeth are closed, the bottom teeth may close in front of the top teeth.

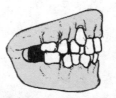

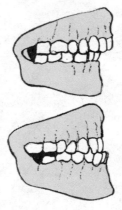

What can I do at home?

- Make sure your child brushes twice and flosses once every day.

- Ask your dentist when your child should stop sucking their thumb or finger or using a pacifier. Sucking a thumb or pacifier can make the top jaw grow too far forward.

- See an **orthodontist** (or-thuh-**don**-tist) if your dentist suggests it. Orthodontists are a special kind of dentist. They are trained to fix crooked teeth and get the teeth and jaw to line up right. Ask your dentist or friends or family for the name of a trusted orthodontist.

When should I call the dentist?

Call the dentist if you think your child may have a bad bite. Your dentist may suggest that you see an orthodontist.

What else should I know?

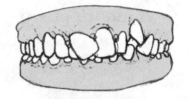

Crooked or crowded teeth can be harder to clean. These teeth may have more problems like cavities and gum disease.

Your dentist may want your child to see an orthodontist at an early age. They can find problems early. That way the problems may be easier to fix.

Some problems don't need to be fixed right away and you can wait. Some children see an orthodontist when they are 7 to 14 years old.

With early treatment the orthodontist can:

- Help the way your child's jaw grows.
- Avoid hurting teeth that stick out.
- Make the teeth look better so your child feels better.
- Help adult teeth come in better.
- Make the child's teeth and lips meet better

Orthodontists often use **braces** to fix crooked teeth and bad bites. Braces are wires that they attach to the teeth for a while. (See page 116.) Your child may also use something called a **retainer**. It guides the way the jaws grow. It also makes more space for the adult teeth to come in through the gums. Kids can take the retainer out when they eat.

Mouth Guard for Sports

What is it?

A **mouth guard** is a soft plastic tray. It fits over the top of teeth and protects your child's mouth from getting hurt.

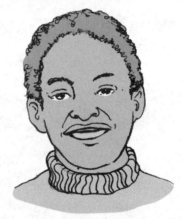

Did you know?

A mouth guard can protect your child from hurting their teeth, lips and tongue. It also can protect their jaw.

It's helpful to wear a mouth guard when you play sports like:

- Basketball
- Baseball
- Football
- Soccer
- Hockey
- Field hockey
- Gymnastics
- Boxing
- Lacrosse
- Volleyball
- Skateboarding
- Scootering
- Bicycling

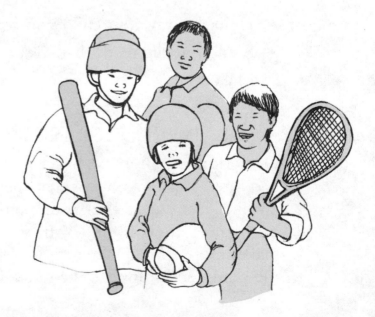

Mouth Guard for Sports

What do I see?

A mouth guard looks like a small curved piece of plastic.

What can I do at home?

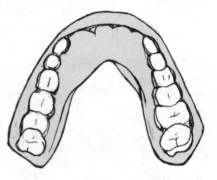

- Buy a "boil and bite" mouth guard from a sporting goods store. Warm water makes it soft. Wait for it too cool, and then have your child put it on their top teeth. As it cools, it hardens into the shape of the teeth and mouth.

- Follow the directions that come with the mouth guard. That way it will fit well and stay in place while playing sports.

- Take care of your child's mouth guard:

- Clean it with cold water before and after use. It can be cleaned with a toothbrush and toothpaste.

- Do not leave a mouth guard in a hot place or in the sun. It could melt and lose its shape.

- Do not let anyone else wear your child's mouth guard. This could spread germs.

- Do not let your child wear someone else's mouth guard. It won't be the right fit and so won't protect your child's mouth. And it can spread germs to them.

- Make sure your child wears a helmet when riding a bike. Helmets are also important when skateboarding, skating, and playing football.

When should I call the dentist?

Call the dentist if you want a mouth guard made for you. This will cost more, but it will fit better than a "boil and bite" guard.

If your child has a mouth guard, take it to show the dentist. The dentist can make sure it is in good shape and fits well.

What else should I know?

The mouth guard should feel good in your child's mouth. They should be able to speak and breathe well with it in.

A mouth guard should be strong and easy to clean.

Because your child in growing and their mouth is changing, the mouth guard should be checked frequently to make sure it still fits well.

Mouth Ulcers
(Canker Sores)

What are they?

An **ulcer** is an open sore. A
mouth ulcer can be on your
lips, cheeks, or tongue. It is
sometimes called a **canker
sore**. Mouth ulcers can be
painful.

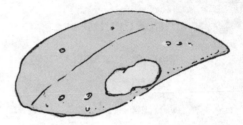

What do I see?

A canker sore is red at first. Then it changes
to a yellow-white color. You may
see one or more in your child's
mouth. The sore lasts 7-14
days.

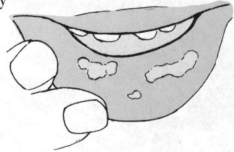

Once it heals you can't see
where it was. There will not
be a scar.

What can I do at home?

- Make sure your child eats and drinks well when they
  have a canker sore. The sores hurt, so children may avoid
  certain food and drinks.
- Choose foods that are mild. Do not give foods that are
  spicy, salty, or have acid in them. Do not give tomatoes
  or oranges to your child when they have sores in their
  mouth. These foods have acid and will cause pain.

Mouth Ulcers (Mouth Sores)

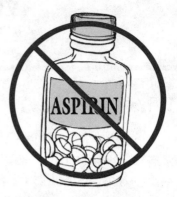

- Give your child Tylenol for pain if you want to. **Do not give your child aspirin**.

When should I call the dentist?

Call the dentist if:

- you see a sore in your child's mouth.
- your child has pain in their mouth.

The dentist may give your child medicine.

What else should I know?

You do not get this mouth sore from someone else. Dentists don't know why people get these sores. They may be from food allergies, stress, poor eating habits, or getting hurt.

After these sores go away, they may come back.

Herpes Simplex Sores

What is it?

Herpes simplex is a germ (virus) that can make a sore on your skin. These sores may be near your mouth or nose. They are also called **cold sores** or **fever blisters**.

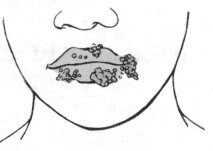

What do I see?

This kind of sore looks like a small, clear blister filled with liquid. They are usually on the face or lip. You may see one blister or a group of them. The skin may itch or tingle before the sore shows up. The blister may break, ooze, and then dry into a scab. After a while the scab falls off and the skin heals. The sore will last for 7-14 days.

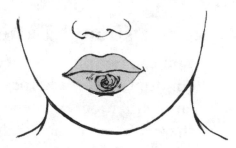

What can I do at home?

- Do not touch the sore or let your child touch it. If you touch it, you can pass the germ to another part of your body or give it to someone else.
- Wash your hands after you touch the sore.

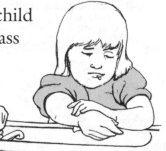

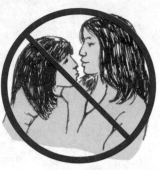

- Do not share forks, spoons, or glasses (cups) with others.
- Do not kiss someone else while you have a sore.
- Do not let someone with a sore kiss you.

When should I call the dentist?

Call the dentist if your child has a sore on their lip or near their mouth.

The dentist may order a medicine to help the sore heal. If you take it right away, the sore may go away faster.

What else should I know?

You can get this type of sore from someone else. Most children who get herpes simplex get it from touching a family member or friend who has it. You can get it if you share a fork, spoon, or drinking glass with someone else who has it. Some people who get this will not get it again. But some people will get more sores. It may be in the same place, or near the same place.

There is no cure for herpes simplex. But new medicines can keep people from getting it again.

Most sores heal in 7-14 days with no scar.

Secondhand Smoke and Children's Teeth

What is it?

Secondhand smoke is the smoke that comes from a burning cigarette, pipe, or cigar. It is also the smoke that a smoker breathes out. If someone near you is smoking, you will breathe in some of their secondhand smoke.

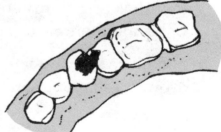

What do I see?

You may see more cavities in the teeth of a child who breathes secondhand smoke. Children who breathe it may cough and wheeze more. They may have more problems with their lungs, like asthma (**as**-ma), bronchitis (brong-kye-tiss) and pneumonia (noo-moh-nyuh).

Second-Hand Smoke and Children's Teeth

What can I do at home?

- Quit smoking. Tell your doctor or dentist that you want help to quit smoking. They have ways to help you quit. There are even some medicines that can help. You can also visit smokefree.gov to get ideas to help you quit.

- Do not smoke near children. If you do smoke, do it outside and away from others.

- Teach your children that smoking or breathing smoke will harm them.

When should I call the dentist?

Tell your dentist if you smoke in the same room as your child.

What else should I know?

Breathing in smoke makes your mouth dry. When your mouth is dry, germs grow faster. This increases your chance of having more cavities.

Nicotine (**nik**-uh-teen) is the drug in tobacco. It lets germs grow in the mouth faster. This makes cavities.

Your Teen's Teeth
(Ages Twelve to Eighteen) 9

Notes

_____

_____

_____

_____

_____

_____

_____

_____

_____

_____

_____

_____

_____

_____

_____

_____

General Care for the Teen's Teeth

What is it?

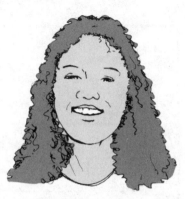

There are some new things to know about caring for your child's teeth when they are older than 12. You have to know how to care for permanent (adult) teeth. You also have to learn about changes that may happen in a teen's life that can affect their teeth and their mouth.

What do I see?

By the age of 12 or 13, most children will have most of their adult teeth.

Sometimes an adult tooth will be missing. Sometimes there may be an extra tooth in the back of their mouth.

What can I do at home?

- Make sure your teen is eating healthy meals and snacks.

- Make sure your teen is getting enough **calcium**. This is extra important for teen girls. Have your teen eat high calcium foods, like cheese, yogurt, and milk. If they don't eat or drink dairy products, ask the doctor or dentist for other ways to get enough calcium.

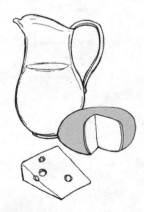

- Try to limit soda. If your teen does drink soda, having one with meals will do less harm to the teeth. It is worse to drink sodas between meals.

- Remind your teen to brush their teeth with a soft toothbrush two times a day, in the morning, and at night before going to bed. Make sure they use toothpaste that has fluoride in it. Be sure they floss once a day.

- Read the information in this chapter about tobacco, body piercing, and eating disorders. Talk to your teen about the problems these things can cause.

When do I call the doctor or dentist?

Call the dentist if:

- your teen still has baby teeth.
- your teen has crooked teeth

Call the doctor if:

- you think your teen may have an eating disorder
- you think your teen is using drugs, or smoking or chewing tobacco

Your teen should see the dentist every 6 months for checkups.

What else should I know?

The teenage years can be an emotional time and busy time. Parents may feel like they spend less time with their teen and have less control over what the teen is doing. It is important to remember to set a good example for your teen, and to continue to guide them. A book that may help is "What to Do For Your Teen's Health." You can buy this book from IHA. Look the back cover of this book to find a phone number and website. You can order the book by phone or online. Your local library may also have a copy of this book you can borrow.

Braces

What is it?

Braces are wires that attach to your teeth. They can fix crooked teeth or a bad bite. A bad bite is when the teeth and jaw do not line up the right way. (See page 100.)

What do I see?

Your teen may have teeth that are uneven, crooked or crowded. The top teeth may stick out too far over the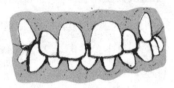
bottom teeth. Or the bottom teeth may be in front of the top teeth when the teeth are together.

What can I do at home?

- Ask your child's dentist if you should take your teen to see an **orthodontist**. This is a special dentist who treats uneven, crooked or crowded teeth. If your child did not see an orthodontist when they were younger, they can see one as a teen.

- Ask your dentist or friends or family for the name of a trusted orthodontist.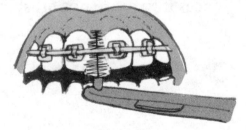

- Make sure your teen does what the orthodontist says: Make sure they use any equipment the dentist gives them.

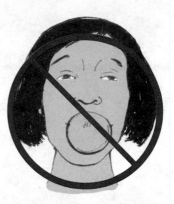

- Brush after every meal and floss at least two times a day.

- Do not eat or chew foods that are sticky, like caramel, peanut brittle, or gum. These foods can bend or break the braces.

- Do not chew ice. Ice can bend or break the braces.

When do I call the dentist?

Call the dentist if any part of your teen's braces breaks. It is very important to have it fixed as soon as possible. (See page 162.)

What else should I know?

Your teen will need to wear a **retainer** after treatment is over. A retainer keeps the teeth in place.

If your teen does not brush and floss well every day while wearing braces, their teeth may have white or yellow-brown spots on them when the braces come off.

They are also more prone to develop cavities while wearing braces if they are not brushing and flossing well.

Back (Wisdom) Teeth

What is it?

Wisdom teeth are the very last teeth in the back of your mouth. They are also known as **third molars**. They are the last adult teeth to come in. Wisdom teeth usually come in between the ages of 16 and 18.

What do I see?

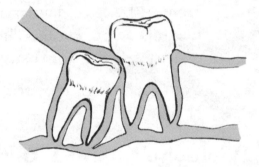

You may or may not see wisdom teeth coming in. Sometimes there is no room for them, because the jaw isn't big enough. If this happens, the teeth may get stuck under the gums. You may see nothing, or you may see only part of the teeth coming in. You may see an infection around these teeth. If there is an infection, you may see puffiness (swelling) near the teeth. You may also see damage to the teeth next to the wisdom teeth. There may be pain, and the jaw may feel stiff.

What can I do at home?

- When your teen is brushing and flossing, be sure they reach the very back of their mouth. This will help keep their wisdom healthy.

- See the dentist if there is pain or swelling. If the wisdom teeth are stuck, you cannot take care of it at home. You must see the dentist.

When should I call the dentist?

Call the dentist if there is pain or swelling in the gums behind the molars.

The dentist will be able to see if there is room for the wisdom teeth to come in. They can also make sure the teeth are healthy. The dentist may decide that the wisdom teeth need to be taken out. They may send your teen to a special dentist called an **oral surgeon** to remove the wisdom teeth

Your teen should see the dentist every six months for a checkup.

What else should I know?

A wisdom tooth that is sideways in the gum is called an **impacted** wisdom tooth. Another problem with wisdom teeth is that a *cyst* (sist) can form around it. A cyst is a small sac filled with liquid. It can harm the bone or other nearby teeth.

If wisdom teeth need to be taken out, do it soon. It is easier to take them out when the person is a teen.

It is common to have impacted wisdom teeth. Many people need to have them taken out.

Eating Problems

What is it?

Eating problems are when teens try to get thin by not eating enough. They may eat very little food, or they may eat a lot and then throw up. There are other types of eating problems, too. Talk to your teen's doctor is you are worried about how they eat.

What do I see?

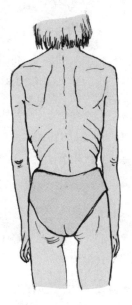

You will see a very, very thin teen who looks like skin and bones. Your teen may be very, very thin but say they are fat. You may notice that a teen barely eats any food. Your teen may always be exercising. Sometimes a teen will eat a lot but go to the bathroom right after to throw up. You may see that a teen eats a lot but never gains weight.

Your teen's mouth may be dry, and they may have a lot of cavities. You may see that the coating of their teeth is wearing away. Teens may have pain in their mouth when they eat hot or cold foods.

What can I do at home?

- Eat healthy foods and exercise. Teach your teen to do the same.

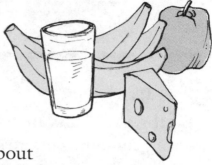

- Serve healthy foods in the right amounts. Teens need to eat three meals and two snacks a day.

- Try to eat meals together as a family.

- Teach your teen to think about food in a healthy way:

  - Don't make your teen eat all the food on their plate. They should stop eating when they are full.

  - Don't use food as a reward.

  - Don't use food to make your teen feel better. When your teen is sad, talk with them. Eating doesn't help.

  - Don't use food to punish your teen.

- Watch for signs that your teen may have an eating problem.

- Don't talk about dieting around your teen. Never tell your teen to go on a diet.

- Notice if your teen goes to the bathroom right after meals.

- Take your teen to the doctor or dentist if you are worried. If you think your teen may have an eating problem, don't believe them when they say it is OK.

- Rinse out their mouth right away if a teen throws up after eating. You can rinse it with water, milk, or water with baking soda in it.

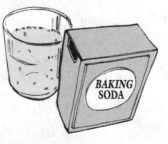

When should I call the doctor or dentist?

Call the doctor if you think your teen has an eating problem. They can tell you where to go for help.

Call the dentist for a checkup if your teen has an eating problem. Eating problems can cause teeth problems, and the dentist can check for these. The dentist may want to do a special fluoride treatment to protect from cavities. If the teen has a dry mouth, the dentist can give them special chewing gum, mouth rinse or toothpaste.

What else should I know?

Eating problems are very serious. Your teen can die from them. They affect the whole body, including the teeth, gums, and mouth.

Eating problems can begin in the early teen years. Any teen can have an eating problem. It doesn't matter if they get all A's in school or are perfect in other ways.

Body Piercing

What is it?

Body piercing is when people make holes in their body for special jewelry. The holes can be almost anywhere including on their skin around the mouth, the lips, or tongue. In the holes, they put rings, studs, and barbells. Body piercing in the mouth can affect your mouth and teeth. It can cause pain, swelling, infection, and drooling. It can also make teeth break or fall out, or the ability to taste. Because of all the bad things that can happen when you have something in your mouth pierced, it should not be done.

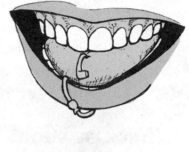

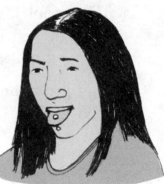

What do I see?

You will see small pieces of metal stuck through holes in or around your teen's mouth area. These can be in the lips, under the bottom lip, or through the tongue. Some are little rings, and some are studs. A **barbell** is worn in a hole through the tongue. It is a stainless steel rod with a ball on each end.

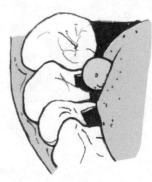

You may see damaged, chipped teeth. This happens when a person bites a barbell by accident, or chews on the jewelry. If a teen has a ring or stud in their lip, you may see damage to their gums.

When a teen has mouth piercings, they may have pain, swelling, infection, or damage to their gums. They may also notice more spit (saliva) flowing in their mouth.

What can I do at home?

- Talk about piercing before your teen decides to do it. Let them know the risks and dangers.

- If you decide to let your teen have a piercing, make sure it is done in a place that is clean and safe.

- Make sure your teen checks the jewelry carefully. Make sure the ball is attached to the bar, and the rings and studs are in place. If a piece gets loose, they could choke on it.

When do I call the dentist?
Call 911 right away if:

- Someone pierces your teen's tongue and there is a lot of bleeding. This can happen if they pierce a blood vessel by accident.

- Your teen's tongue swells up and they have trouble breathing. In extreme cases, the tongue can get so swollen it can close the airway and stop the person's breathing. Your teen could die from this.

Call the dentist if:

- Your teen has pain or swelling in their mouth near the piercing.

- You see a chipped tooth or damage to their gums.

Have the dentist check your teen's mouth after a piercing. They can make sure there is no infection. If there is an infection, the dentist may want to give your teen some medicine.

Smokeless Tobacco

What is it?

Smokeless tobacco is made of the same stuff that's in cigarettes. But instead of smoking it, you put it right into your mouth. Some kinds are sniffed into your nose. **Chewing tobacco** and **snuff** are the two main types. Smokeless tobacco can cause cancer in the mouth.

What do I see?

Chewing tobacco comes in a packet or a small can. A person will put some of this in their mouth and chew it up. It mixes with the spit (saliva) to make a wad. You may see this wad in someone's mouth. Or you may see a white or yellow-brown patch, or a thick wrinkled area.

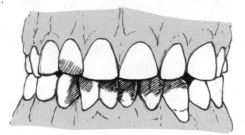

You may see that the person's teeth are stained. They may have bad breath. You may see their gums pull back (recede) from their teeth. This makes the teeth look longer because you can see the roots. You may see cavities on these roots. Roots that you can see may hurt from hot or cold foods and drinks. Chewing tobacco has sugar in it and so people who use it often have more cavities.

What can I do at home?

- Get help from a doctor or dentist if your teen is chewing tobacco. They have ways to help people quit.

- Notice if your teen has a patch or wrinkled area in their mouth. If it is from chewing tobacco, it could become cancer.

When should I call the dentist?

Call the dentist if you see wrinkles or a spot where the tobacco sits. If the dentist can check the spots early, they may not become cancer.

Call the dentist if you see bleeding or receding gums.

What else should I know?

Smokeless tobacco and snuff can cause mouth cancer. Both contain nicotine. The nicotine is released when you chew the tobacco. Your teen can get addicted to **nicotine** very quickly.

There will be more cavities on the side where the tobacco sits in the mouth.

People who chew tobacco can begin to lose their senses of taste and smell.

Smoking Tobacco

What is it?

Tobacco is a kind of plant. People often smoke tobacco in cigarettes, cigars, or pipes.

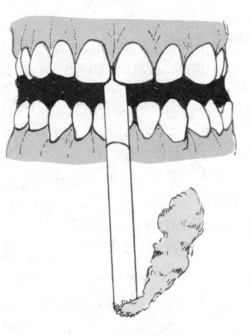

What do I see?

You will see many people who start to smoke, starting in their teenage years.

You may see gum disease. People who smoke have more gum disease.

What can I do at home?

• Talk to your teen about smoking. Make sure they know all about the health risks, including the harm it does to their mouth and teeth. (See the facts on the next page.)

• Help your child quit smoking. Ask their doctor or dentist for help.

When do I call the dentist?

Tell the dentist if your teen is smoking. Ask the dentist to give your teen information about smoking and to help them quit.

Smoking Tobacco

What else should I know?

It is very easy to become addicted to smoking. Even teens can quickly become addicted. It is very hard to quit, and so your teen will need a lot of support.

Sometimes knowing a certain fact can change a person's mind about smoking. Here are some facts you can share when you talk with your teen:

- Smoking causes wrinkles to form when you are younger.
- The longer you smoke, the more likely you are to get sick from it.
- People who smoke have a greater chance of having mouth, throat, lung, and other cancers.

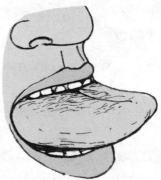

- If you smoke and drink alcohol, you have a very high risk for mouth cancer.
- Cigars also cause mouth cancer.
- Cigarette smokers can get a hairy black tongue.
- Smokers lose their teeth from gum disease.
- If you quit smoking, many of the bad effects will get better.

Adults

10

Notes

_____

_____

_____

_____

_____

_____

_____

_____

_____

_____

_____

_____

_____

_____

Fillings

What is it?

The dentist uses a dental filling to fix teeth. It fills in holes (cavities), or parts of the teeth that are worn down, or hurt. There are several types of fillings that may be used.

What do I see?

You may see a silver patch on the tooth. Or you may see a patch that's almost the same color as the tooth.

What can I do at home?

- Brush your teeth twice a day and floss your teeth once a day. This helps prevent cavities so you don't need fillings.
- Use toothpaste with fluoride in it.

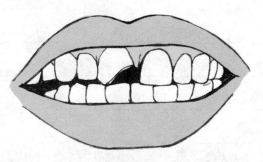

When should I call the dentist?

Call the dentist if:

- your tooth breaks.
- your tooth hurts when you have sweet, hot, or cold foods.

- your new filling feels "high." This means it touches the tooth above it before your other teeth come together when you close your mouth.

See the dentist for a checkup every 6 months to make sure you don't need a filling.

What else should I know?

Most fillings are done in one visit. If you need more than 2 or 3 fillings, you may have to come back for a second visit.

Hot and cold things may bother your tooth for a few days or weeks after you have a filling.

There are different types of dental fillings. Your dentist will talk to you about what kind is best for you.

- **Silver fillings** look like the color silver.

- **Composite fillings** are a mix of plastic and other things. They are the same color as your tooth.

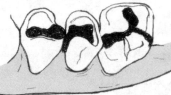

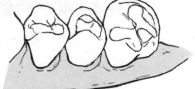

- **Glass ionomers** are like composite fillings, but they have a small amount of fluoride in them. The fluoride comes out slowly. It helps stop the tooth from getting a new cavity.

Missing Teeth

What is it?

This is when there is a space in your mouth, because a tooth has fallen out or never came in. A tooth can get knocked out by an injury. Or it could fall out because of tooth decay or gum disease. Dentists can replace missing teeth.

Did you know?

You should replace missing teeth to keep your mouth healthy. When there is a space from a missing tooth, the other teeth may shift. This will mean that your bite may be off.

Missing teeth can be replaced by:

- A partial denture that you can take out
- A full denture
- A bridge
- An implant

You can learn about each of these later in this chapter.

What do I see?

You will see a space in your mouth where the tooth was. Your face may sag on the outside in that spot. If you are missing back teeth, your front teeth may stick out and have spaces between them.

Missing Teeth

The teeth near the space may tilt in toward it. The gums around these tilted teeth may be swollen. Your gums may bleed when you floss your teeth.

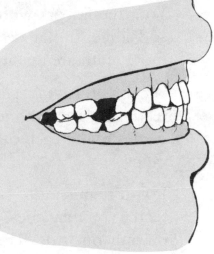

What can I do at home?

- Brush your teeth twice a day and floss once a day.
- Use toothpaste with fluoride in it.
- Eat the right foods. (See page 45.)
- See the dentist every 6 months for checkups.

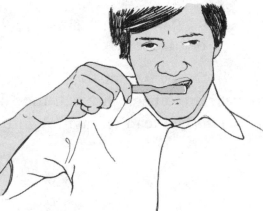

When should I call the dentist?

Call the dentist if:

- You lose an adult tooth.
- If you have missing teeth and want to replace them.

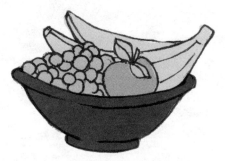

What else should I know?

Your teeth work with each other to help you chew, speak, and smile. It may be hard to do these things when one or more teeth are missing.

When you have a space where your missing tooth was, the teeth near it often move around. This changes the way your teeth fit with each other. It can put stress on your teeth and gums.

If you're missing teeth, you may chew on only one side. This can put stress on your jaw joints. This can cause pain in your jaw or headaches.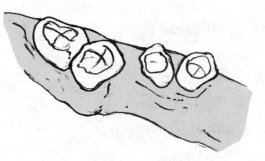

It can be harder to clean your teeth when they move or when they're crooked. This can lead to cavities and gum disease.

Crown

What is it?

A **crown** is a treatment for a broken or damaged tooth. It may also be called a **cap**. A crown is placed over the damaged tooth. It makes your tooth the right shape and size again. A crown can be made of metal, porcelain, or both. Porcelain is a hard white material that is also used to make sinks, tiles or dishes.

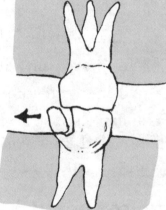

What do I see?

You may see that you have a tooth that is cracked or badly broken. Or may have pain from hot or cold foods, or when you bite down on something. It may mean that you need a crown. You may want to get a crown if your front teeth are poorly shaped or don't look white. A crown made of porcelain will look like a real tooth.

Crown

What can I do at home?

- Treat your crowned teeth like your real teeth. Brush your teeth twice a day and floss them once a day. Use toothpaste with fluoride in it.

- Do not chew sticky foods or hard foods like ice, hard candy or peanut brittle if you have a porcelain crown. The crown can break or come loose.

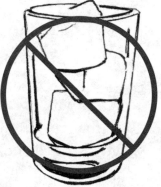

When should I call the dentist?

Call the dentist right away if:

- Your tooth breaks.
- You have pain when you bite down.
- Your crown comes off.

You can also ask your dentist about a crown if you're not happy with how your front teeth look. Tell the dentist how you want them to look.

What else should I know?

The dentist can help you decide which crown is best for you. Metal crowns are stronger than porcelain crowns. A metal crown can go on your back teeth where it doesn't show. A crown with porcelain and metal can go on front or back teeth.

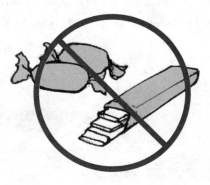

Crown

On the first visit the dentist will get your tooth ready for a crown. You will get a plastic, **temporary crown** that will be on your teeth for a short time. Ask if you should floss around temporary crown. Do not chew gum or sticky candy when you have a temporary crown. On the next visit the dentist will put in the **permanent crown**. This is the one you will have for a long time. You should be able to floss between teeth with a permanent crown and the teeth next to them.

If your temporary crown comes off, the dentist may glue it on again or make a new one. If you don't go to the dentist, the teeth around your lost crown could move. Then your permanent crown may not fit.

A new crown should feel good in a few days. Tell the dentist if you bite down and feel the crown first. The dentist can make it fit better.

Bridge

What is it?

A **bridge** replaces one or more missing teeth. To make it, the dentist files down the two teeth on either side of the missing one. Then they attach a single piece of porcelain with the false tooth (or teeth) in it. This piece of porcelain also has two crowns in it that connect to the teeth on either side of the missing one(s).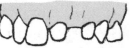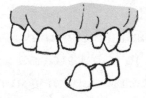

Did you know?

You cannot take your bridge out. Only a dentist can do that.

A bridge helps to keep the normal shape of your face. It can help to hold up your lips and cheeks.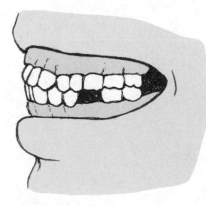

What do I see?

You will see a space between your teeth before you get the bridge. After the bridge is in place it will look like real teeth.

Bridge

What can I do at home?

- Brush your teeth twice a day and floss your teeth every day. Use toothpaste with fluoride in it.

- Use a floss threader. (See picture) This helps you get the floss between your bridge and gums.

When should I call the dentist?

Call the dentist if:

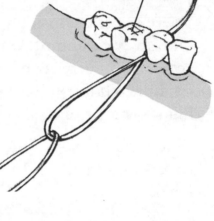

Bridge

- you are missing a tooth and want it replaced.

- you have pain in the bridge area. You may need a new bridge if there are problems with the teeth or gums under it.

See the dentist every 6 months for a checkup.

What else should I know?

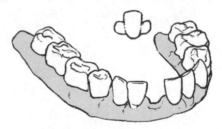

- Your dentist will talk to you about the best bridge for you.

- Bridges are made from metals like gold or other alloys.

- Porcelain can be used to make the bridge look like natural teeth.

Root Canal

What is it?

A **root canal** is something a dentist can do to fix a tooth with deep decay.

Did you know?

There is a space inside your teeth called the **pulp**. It has blood vessels and nerves in it. The pulp can get infected if you have a deep cavity or a crack in your tooth. It can also get infected if you get hit in the face. If there are many fillings on the same tooth, it can get infected.

When the pulp gets infected, you need a root canal. You can have a lot of pain and swelling in your face if the tooth isn't fixed.

The infection can cause a fever. It can spread to other parts of your body.

What do I see?

You may not see anything wrong, but have pain in your teeth or gums. It may hurt when you bite down on food. It may hurt when you eat or drink something hot or cold. The pain may stay even after you take the food away from your teeth. The gum around your tooth may hurt when you touch it.

You may see a sore on your gum with pus in it. You may see a tooth that is gray in color. Your face may be puffy.

Root Canal

What can I do at home?

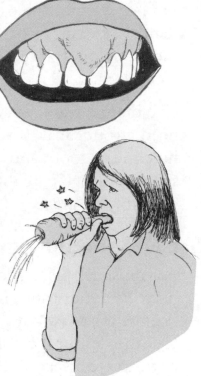

- Take care of your teeth. This can prevent you from needing a root canal.

- Brush your teeth with a soft toothbrush2 times a day. Floss between your teeth every day.

- Use toothpaste with fluoride in it.

- See the dentist for checkups every 6 months.

- Do what the dentist tells you to do after a root canal. Take Tylenol or the pain medicine your dentist gave you if you have pain. And take other medicine that the dentist may have ordered to prevent or treat infection.

When should I call the dentist?

Call the dentist if:

- you have a dull ache and pressure in your upper teeth or jaw.

- your tooth hurts when you bite into food.

- your tooth hurts when you eat or drink hot or cold things.

- it feels like your heart is beating in your tooth.

- the pain in your tooth wakes you up.

Do not wait for the pain to go away before you call the dentist. It won't go away. The tooth will start to hurt even more. If you wait too long, the dentist may have to pull the tooth out.

The dentist will take an X-ray of your tooth to see if you need a root canal. If you do, the dentist will drill a small hole in the tooth and clean the nerve space (pulp). **The tooth and the roots will stay in place.**

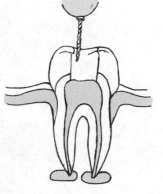

What else should I know?

For most people, a root canal does not hurt. But your tooth may hurt or feel strange for a few days after a root canal. Call the dentist if it still hurts. You may need to see a special dentist called an **endodontist**. These dentists only do root canals. Your dentist will tell you if you need to see an endodontist.

If your tooth has a crack, the dentist may ask you not to grind your teeth or chew hard things like ice.

If you have a root canal, do not chew or bite on the tooth until the dentist puts a crown over it. If the crown is not put on, your tooth can break. If it breaks into pieces, the tooth may need to get pulled out. Most of the time, it is better to have a root canal than to have the tooth pulled.

Removable Partial Dentures ("Partials")

What is it?

Removable partial dentures are false teeth that you can put in and take out yourself. They replace missing teeth. A set is sometimes called a **partial**. A partial helps you chew and speak. Like a bridge, it supports your lips and cheeks.

What do I see?

A partial has false teeth hooked to a plastic base. The base is the color of your gums. It has metal clasps that will hold the partial onto your real teeth.

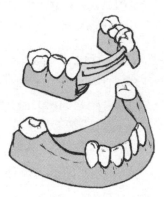

What can I do at home?

- Get used to taking the partial in and out. It should fit in place easily. Never force it to fit. You may bend or break a clasp. You may hurt the teeth that hold it in place.

- Be careful when you eat at first. Start with soft foods cut in small pieces. Chew on both sides of your mouth. Try not to eat sticky or hard foods as you get used to the partial. It should feel good to eat once the partial fits right.

Removable Partial Dentures

- Get used to speaking with the partial. If you can't speak clearly at first, practice by reading out loud. Repeat words that are hard to say. Once you are used to it, the partial should help you to talk clearly.

- Clean your partial every day:

  1. Put something soft under it while you clean it (like a towel at the sink). That way, if you drop it you won't break it.

  2. Take it out and rinse it first.

  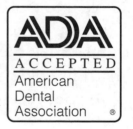

  3. Then use a soft, wet toothbrush to clean it. This keeps it from getting stained and dirty. There are special brushes for your partial.

  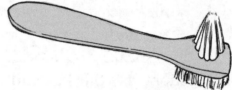

  4. Use hand soap or mild dish soap to clean it. Or use a denture cleaner. Make sure it has the American Dental Association (ADA) Seal of Acceptance on it.

  5. Then rinse it very well.

- Clean your real teeth next to the partial with toothpaste. Germs can get stuck on the metal clasps that touch your real teeth. These teeth are more likely to get cavities.

When should I call the dentist?

Call the dentist if:

- You have a problem with your partial.
- The partial puts too much force on one area. That area feels sore.
- Your partial breaks or chips or feels rough. Do not try to fix it yourself.
- A tooth or hook comes off the partial.

What else should I know?

Your dentist should tell you when to wear your partial and when to take it out. They may want you to wear it during the day and take it out at night. Your dentist can also show you how to clean your partial.

If you don't keep your partial wet, it can change shape and not fit well. Put it in a glass of water or denture cleanser while you sleep. Change this water or cleanser each day. Brush and rinse your partial before you put it back in your mouth.

Your mouth can change as you get older, or if you gain or lose weight. Your gums can shrink. This leaves a space between your gums and the partial. The dentist will need to fix it.

Dentures

What is it?

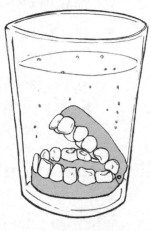

Dentures are a set of false teeth attached to a plastic base. It can replace your top teeth, bottom teeth, or both. It also supports your cheeks and lips. Your face can sag and look older if you don't wear it.

What do I see?

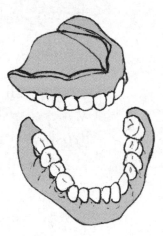

The plastic base is the color of your gums. The upper denture base covers the roof of your mouth. The lower denture base looks like a horseshoe. It's shaped that way so there is room for your tongue. The teeth in dentures look like natural healthy teeth.

What can I do at home?

- Get used to eating with dentures
- Start with soft foods cut into small pieces.
- Chew slowly on both sides of your mouth. This way, the dentures don't move around.
- Don't try to bite things with your front teeth. When you have dentures, you must use your back teeth for all the chewing.

- Get used to speaking with your dentures. If you can't speak clearly at first, practice by reading out loud. Repeat words that are hard to say.

- Take out your dentures and clean them every day.

- Clean them after meals and before you go to bed.

- Use a soft brush to clean them so they don't stain.

- Put a towel below you when you take the dentures out. That way they won't break if you drop them.

- Brush your gums and tongue with a soft brush, even though you have no teeth.

- Keep your dentures away from small children and pets. Dogs may chew on them.

When should I call the dentist?

Call the dentist if:

- you get sore spots in your mouth. The dentures may need to be fixed.

- the dentures feel loose. Your dentist may want you to use a cream to hold it in place. Call 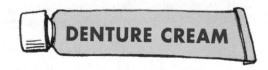 your dentist if the cream doesn't help. You may get a sore spot.

See the dentist every year for checkups, even though you don't have teeth. They can make sure your mouth is healthy and that your dentures still fit well. Ask your dentist to check for diseases like cancer of the mouth.

Dentures

What else should I know?

Dentures usually should be out of your mouth at least 4 hours a day. Ask your dentist how long you should wear your dentures each day. Your dentist may want you to wear them all the time at first. That way you can get used to them. Then, once you are used to the dentures, your dentist may want you to take them out at night.

Dentures may feel loose when you first come home with them. Your cheeks and gums learn to hold them in place. A seal is made between the spit in your mouth and your gums.

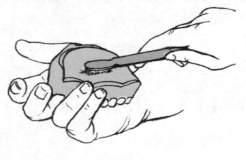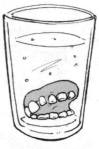

A denture can slip if you yawn, laugh, cough, or smile. Bite down and swallow to get it back in place.

Dentures wear out with time. They may not fit right if you gain or lose weight. Dentures that don't fit right can cause problems. Do not try to fix them yourself. Let the dentist fix them. They may need to be replaced. Or they may need to be **relined**. That's when the dentist puts new plastic under them for a better fit.

Jaw Pain

What is it?

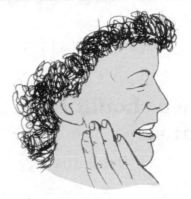

Pain in your face, neck, or shoulders can start in your jaws. It can happen when you grind your teeth or clench them together.

What do I see?

You may feel pain but not see anything else. You may have pain when you move your lower jaw. You may not be able to open your mouth very wide. You may have headaches, earaches, or ringing in your ears. You may wake up with sore teeth, muscles, or jaw.

You won't know if you grind your teeth when you sleep. Often a family member hears it. It sounds like you are chewing on rocks.

What can I do at home?

- See the dentist or doctor if you have pain in your jaw. They can find out what is causing it.

- Follow these tips to help your jaw pain. Your dentist or doctor may suggest other things to do.

  - Eat soft foods
  - Put ice or heat packs on your jaw: 5 minutes, 3 times a day.
  - Hold your jaw in place when you yawn.

- Don't chew gum.
- Do exercises for the joints and muscles in your jaws.

When should I call the dentist?

Call the dentist if:

• you have pain in your jaws.

• it's hard to open or close your mouth.

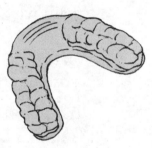

The dentist may order medicine for you. It will relax your jaw muscles or help with your pain.

What else should I know?

If you grind or clench your teeth, it can wear them down and give you jaw pain. It can make your teeth crack or break. The dentist may want to make a plastic **bite plate** for you. It fits in your mouth and stops you from grinding your teeth when you sleep.

If a doctor or dentist says you need surgery for jaw pain, ask another doctor as well. This is called a second opinion.

Dry Mouth

What is it?

Dry mouth is when you don't have enough spit (saliva) to keep your mouth wet.

Did you know?

Everyone has a dry mouth once in a while. It can happen when you are nervous or upset, or when you are sick. But if you have dry mouth a lot, it can cause problems. You can get lots of cavities in your teeth. This can happen fast.

What do I see?

Your lips may look dry and cracked. They may bleed. Your tongue may be dry. You may have mouth sores.

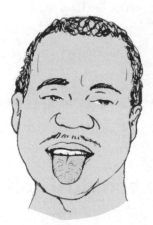

What can I do at home?

- Take good care of your teeth to prevent cavities. With a dry mouth you can get cavities very fast.

  - Brush your teeth at least twice a day and floss your teeth every day.
  - Use toothpaste with fluoride in it.
  - Use a mouthwash with fluoride in it. Make sure the mouthwash that you use does not have alcohol in it.
  - Brush your teeth right away if you eat sticky foods.

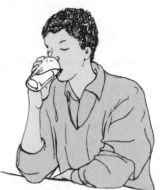

- Use a gel that is made for people who have a dry mouth. Your dentist can tell you which one to use. Or ask at the drugstore.

- Sip water often.

- Sip water when you eat. This will make it easier to chew and swallow.

- Don't drink things with caffeine. These include coffee, tea and most sodas. Caffeine can dry out your mouth.

- Don't use tobacco and alcohol. They can make your mouth dry.

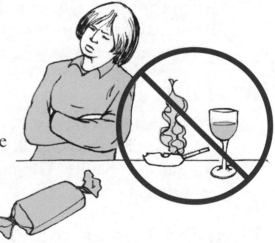

- Suck on candy with no sugar. This helps to make more spit in your mouth.

- Don't eat spicy or salty foods if it hurts to eat them.

When should I call the dentist?

Call the dentist if you think you have dry mouth.

Your dentist may want to give you medicine to make your spit glands work better. They may get you toothpaste with extra fluoride in it.

Or they may give you a gel to help keep your mouth wet.

See the dentist every 6 months for a checkup.

What else should I know?

The spit in your mouth is important. Spit is also called **saliva**. It's made from the **saliva glands** in your mouth. When these glands don't work well, you get dry mouth.

Spit helps you digest your food. It protects your mouth from germs that cause infections. If you don't have enough spit, you may get infections in your mouth. Spit helps your teeth so they don't get cavities in them.

Some medicines for high blood pressure or depression can give you a dry mouth. You can also get dry mouth from diseases like Diabetes, Parkinson's or HIV/AIDS.

Saliva glands can get hurt from radiation treatment for cancer. Some medicines for cancer give you a dry mouth. Hurting your head or neck can harm the nerves that tell your glands to make spit.

Emergencies

11

Notes

_____
_____
_____
_____
_____
_____
_____
_____
_____
_____
_____
_____
_____
_____

Knocked-out Teeth

What is it?

A whole tooth may get knocked out of your mouth if you hit your face hard on something. It mostly happens to the front teeth.

What do I see?

You will see a space where the tooth was. You may see blood in the space. You may see the tooth on the ground or in your mouth.

What can I do at home?

- Call the dentist right away. Say you have an emergency. Fast action can save your tooth.

- Try to find the tooth that came out.

- Do not touch the root of the tooth. The root is the part that is normally inside your gum. Hold the tooth only by the end that you chew with.

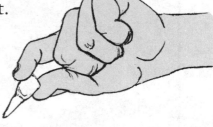

- If you find the tooth, gently rinse it with salt water or cool tap water. Do not use soap. Do not rub or scrub the tooth to get dirt off it.

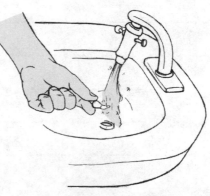

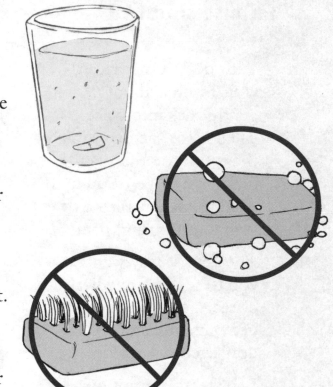

- Holding the tooth by the end you chew with, gently replace it in the socket (hole it came out of). If you cannot replace it, put the tooth in a cup of milk or your saliva (spit).

- Get to the dentist right away.

- Keep the tooth wet.

If it's a baby tooth:

- Put a clean, folded cloth or gauze over the bleeding. Make sure the child can't choke on it.

- Have the child bite gently on the gauze or cloth for 15 minutes.

- Call the dentist if there is still bleeding after 15 minutes.

When should I call the dentist or doctor?

Call the dentist right away if your tooth comes out. If the office is closed, call the dentist's emergency number.

See the dentist within 30 minutes of your tooth coming out. That way there is a good chance it can be put back into your mouth and saved.

What else should I know?

Your dentist may clean your tooth and put it gently back into place. Then he or she may attach the tooth to other teeth to make it stronger. You may need to take medicine to stop infection and pain.

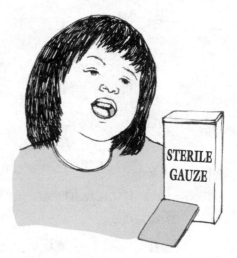

The dentist may want you to see your medical doctor. You may need to get a tetanus shot so you don't get sick.

Baby teeth are not put back into the mouth when they get knocked out.

Adults and children should wear a mouth guard on their teeth when they play sports.

STERILE GAUZE

Chipped or Broken Teeth

What is it?

It's when part of your tooth breaks off. You can break your teeth if you get hit hard in the face, like in an accident. You can also chip or break a tooth if you eat something hard like ice or hard candy. It can also happen if you have a big cavity.

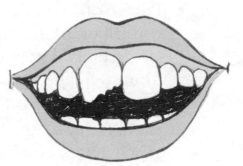

Did you know?

A tooth with a hole in it can break like an eggshell. A tooth can chip or break if it has been fixed with a filling. This can happen when you bite something hard or grind your teeth.

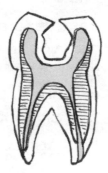

What do I see?

If your tooth has a small break, you will see some of the tooth missing. But sometimes the tooth may not look broken. You may just feel a sharp edge when your tongue touches the spot. Your tongue could get sore if you can't stop it from touching the spot.

If most of the tooth breaks off, you may see a space where the tooth was. Only the root may be left.

What can I do at home?

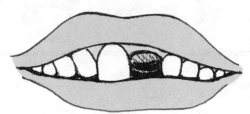

- Call the dentist.

- Rinse the area with warm water to clean it.

- Put ice on your face if you fell or got hit in the face. This will stop it from swelling.

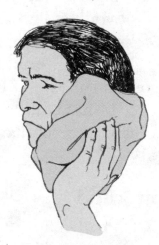

- Hold gauze or a paper towel firmly on the hurt area if you're bleeding. Do not press right on the tooth. Just press on the gums.

- Take the broken tooth with you to the dentist, if you have it. The dentist will try to save the tooth.

- Do not take aspirin.

- Do not put any medicine on the tooth or gums.

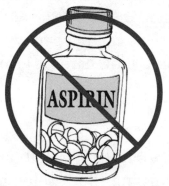

Chipped or Broken Teeth

When should I call the dentist?

Call the dentist right away if you chip or break a tooth.

The dentist can tell you if you have to come in right away. If it's a small break, it may be okay to wait until your normal visit. If it's a big break, you may need to see the dentist right away.

What else should I know?

For a small break, the dentist may just need to smooth the tooth or put in a filling. For a big break, you may need a crown. The dentist may need to do a root canal if the inside of the tooth is hurt. If the tooth can't be fixed, the dentist may need to pull it.

If you hurt your back teeth, one of the top points may break off. Or there may be a deep crack. If the crack is in the nerve space, your dentist will do a root canal and a crown. You may have a lot of pain if the nerve is showing.

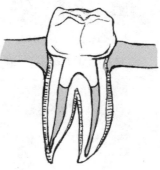

Broken Braces

What is it?

Braces are used to fix a bad bite or crooked teeth. (See page 116.) Braces are made of brackets and wires. These wires can break or get loose. Then they can cut your gums, cheeks, or lips.

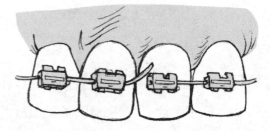

What do I see?

You may see a wire or other part that sticks out. It may cut your lips, cheeks, or gums.

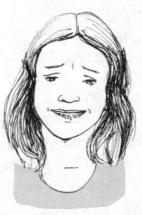

What can I do at home?

- Use wax from your orthodontist to cover the wire or bracket.
- Do not try to take the wire or bracket off.
- Don't chew gum or sticky candy if you have braces.
- Do not eat hard food like ice and hard candy.

Broken Braces

When should I call the orthodontist?

Call the orthodontist right away if part of your braces are broken or loose.

They will tell you if you should go to the office. It may not be urgent if the broken part does not bother you. But you could choke if a piece comes off in your mouth. Let the orthodontist decide what you should do.

What else should I know?

The orthodontist may tell you to cut the wire very close to the brace with a nail clipper. If you can't do this, you should put wax on it.

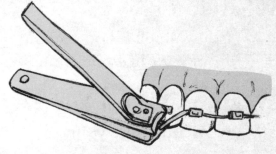

A brace or wire can break if you eat foods that are too hard or sticky.

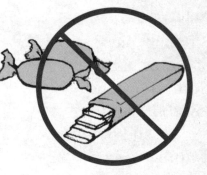

Biting the Lips, Cheeks, or Tongue

What is it?

Your teeth can bite into your lips, cheeks, or tongue. This can happen when you fall or have an accident.

What do I see?

You will see blood coming from your lips or tongue.

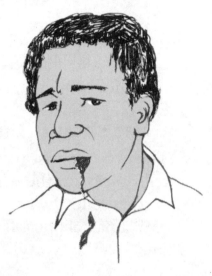

What can I do at home?

- Gently rinse your mouth with cool water.

- Bite on a piece of **gauze**, a clean cloth, or a paper towel. Hold it on the cut and press it firmly to stop the bleeding.

- Gently pull your tongue forward (like you're sticking it out) if it's bleeding. Press gauze or cloth firmly on your tongue.

164

Biting the Lips, Cheeks, or Tongue

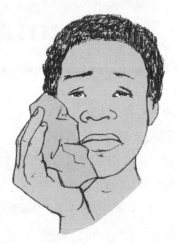

- Put ice on your lips or cheek if there is swelling. Wrap ice in a towel. This is called a **cold compress**. Put it on the cut.

When should I call the dentist or doctor?

Call the dentist or doctor right away if you have a cut that is bleeding a lot. Say you have an emergency.

Go to the emergency room right away if:

- you can't stop the bleeding and can't reach your dentist.
- you fall and hit your head hard.
- you break your jaw. Your jaw could be broken if your teeth don't fit together when you close your mouth.

What else should I know?

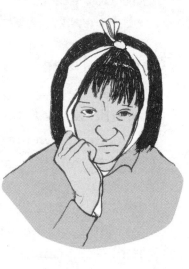

The dentist may want to see you right away if your cut still bleeds after you press gauze on it for 15 minutes.

The dentist may want you to see an **oral surgeon**. An oral surgeon is a dentist who can do surgery. They can fix big problems in your mouth. The oral surgeon may want to use stitches to close the cut so it heals faster.

Dental Cellulitis

What is it?

Dental cellulitis (sell-you-lye-tis) is an infection of the mouth. You can get this if you have problems in your mouth and do not see a dentist to fix them. This is a very bad disease and needs to be treated by a dentist.

You could die from it if you do not get help right away.

What do I see?

Your face swells up on the side of the infection. Swelling may go all the way to your eyes. It may go to your neck. The swelling can be so bad it makes your face look bad.

You may have a bad toothache.

Dental Cellulitis

What can I do at home?

- Call the dentist right away or go to the hospital emergency room (ER).

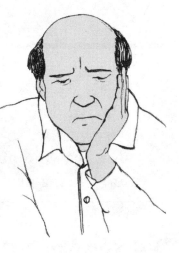

When should I call the dentist?

Call the dentist right away if you have a bad toothache or swelling in your face. You may be able to stop the infection if you call right away.

Go to the emergency room right away if you can't reach your dentist.

What else should I know?

Swelling around your face can be dangerous. If the swelling is near your eye, it can go to your brain. If it's near your neck, it can stop you from breathing.

If you have an infection, you must see the dentist to get it treated. If you don't treat it, it can turn into dental cellulitis.

These are things that can cause an infection in your mouth:

- Gum disease
- A large hole in your tooth or gum
- A pierced tongue (See page 123.)
- The dentist may want you to see an **oral surgeon**. This is a special dentist who can fix bad problems in your mouth.

Pericoronitis

What is it?

Pericoronitis
(pair-ee- ko-ro-nye-tus)
is when your gums swell
up when a new tooth is
coming in. This is painful.

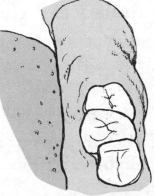

Did you know?

It happens when germs
or food get stuck in your
gums. They get stuck under the
flap of gum that covers the tooth
that is coming in. It often happens
to the bottom **18-year molars**.
These are called **wisdom teeth**.
(See page 118.)

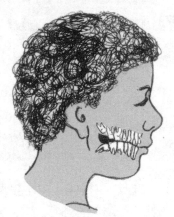

What do I see?

The flap of gum may get
very puffy. It may hurt
when you touch it. The
area may get so puffy that
it hurts if you touch under
your jaw. The pain in your
mouth may feel like it's
going to your head. It may
also be hard to breathe.

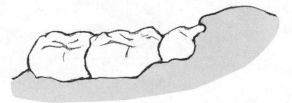

Pericoronitis

You may see **pus** (yellow-green liquid) come from the puffy spot. It may taste bad.

What can I do at home?

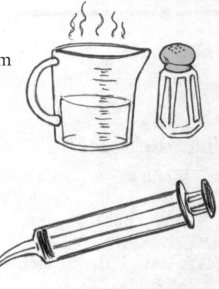

- Rinse your mouth with warm salt water. Make sure the water is not so hot it burns your mouth. Use 1/2 cup water and 1/2 teaspoon salt. Do this three times a day.

- Use a special tool that the dentist gives you. It works like a turkey baster to clean and rinse the area. You squirt water under the flap of gum that hurts.

When should I call the dentist?

Call the dentist right away if your gums swell up or hurt. Say you have an emergency.

The dentist will decide if you need to come to the office. They will clean your gums, and may give you medicine to keep the swelling down.

What else should I know?

If you have a painful bottom gum, it can get worse if the top tooth touches it. It can happen again unless the dentist fixes the problem.

If a wisdom tooth is causing the problem, the dentist may have to take it out.

Food Stuck Between the Teeth

What is it?

Food can get stuck between your teeth. It can give you a toothache.

What do I see?

You may see swelling between 2 teeth. You may see nothing but feel pain. It may hurt when you touch the gums around your teeth.

What can I do at home?

- Use dental floss to try to get the food out. Be gentle.
- Never use a sharp tool to take out food that is stuck.
- Never use a pin or a needle. These things may hurt your gums.

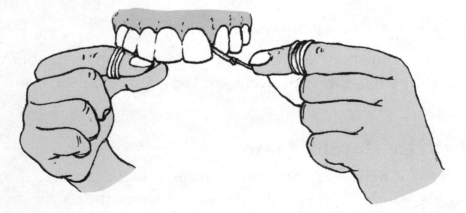

Food Stuck Between the Teeth

When should I call the dentist?

Call the dentist if you can't get the food out after 2 days.

The dentist will try to get it out with floss. But if that doesn't work, they can use special tools to clean between your teeth.

What else should I know?

Never put aspirin or other pain medicine on your gums near the tooth that hurts. It can burn your gums.

Popcorn kernels often get stuck between teeth. Use floss to remove the popcorn kernels.

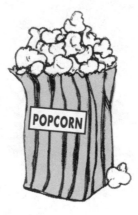

Illness and Your Teeth 12

Notes

_____

_____

_____

_____

_____

_____

_____

_____

_____

_____

_____

_____

_____

_____

Illness and Your Teeth

What is it?

Some illnesses may increase your chance of having bad teeth and gum problems. Examples are being **obese** or having **diabetes**. If you are **obese**, it means you are too heavy for your height. If you have **diabetes**, it means you have too much sugar in your blood.

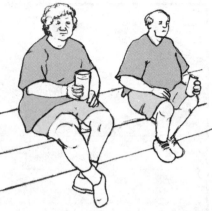

Did you know?

If you are obese:

• you may get puffy or bleeding gums.

• you are more likely to get diabetes.

If you have diabetes:

• you can get bad gum disease.

• you can lose the bone that holds your teeth in place.

• you may get a dry mouth.

• you may get more cavities.

What can I do at home?

Take care of your body. This can prevent you from getting these illnesses.

• Eat foods that are good for you. (See page 45.)

• Exercise or stay active.

- See your doctor for checkups every year.
- Do what your doctor tells you to stay healthy.
- Keep your body at a healthy weight. If you are too heavy, lose weight. Ask your doctor for help.

Take care of your teeth.

- Brush your teeth at least twice a day, and floss your teeth every day.
- Brush and floss after snacks and meals too.
- See the dentist every 6 months for a checkup.

When should I call the dentist?

Call the dentist if:

- your doctor says you are obese
- your doctor says you have diabetes
- you think you have gum disease
- you have pain in your teeth or gums

See the dentist for a checkup every 6 months.

What else should I know?

There are many illnesses that can cause problems for your teeth and gums. With some illnesses it is hard to know if you are sick. If you have regular checkups with your doctor, you can find out if you have an illness. And if you know about it early on, you can take better care of yourself.

You may not know if you have diabetes. There may not be any clear symptoms. Your doctor can give you a test if it seems you might have it. If you have diabetes it is very important to get treated right away.

Losing weight and eating right are very important. You can stop yourself from getting obese if you try. You have control of this. If you are overweight, you are too heavy. If you are obese, you are **much** too heavy. So if you are overweight, use this as a warning. Lose weight before you get obese.

Gum disease and obesity could give you more chance of getting these diseases:

- Heart attack
- Stroke
- High blood pressure
- Some kinds of cancer
- Diabetes

Other Infections

What is it?

Infections are sicknesses caused by germs. You can get different kinds of infections in your mouth. Your dentist needs to look at your mouth to know what kind it is and how to treat it. Some infections happen more often to small children. Others are more common in adults.

What do I see?

Your gums may look puffy, red, or gray. They may bleed or hurt when you press them. You may see sores in your mouth, filled with yellow or white liquid.

You may have trouble swallowing and speaking. You may also have bad breath. Sometimes you have a fever as high as 104 degrees F°. Children may have a headache or be fussy.

What can I do at home?

- Do as the dentist tells you. They may tell you to rinse your mouth out with something.
- You may need to have a liquid diet for a few days.

When do I call the dentist?

Call the dentist if:

- your mouth hurts
- you see sores in your mouth
- you see any changes in your gums

Other Infections

What else should I know?

Some infections are **contagious**. That means you can pass them on to someone else. Your dentist will tell you if you have an infection, and what kind it is. They will also tell you how to treat it, and how long it will take to go away. Do what your dentist tells you to do to get rid of the infection.

Your dentist may give you a kind of medicine called an **antibiotic**. It kills the germs that cause infection.

If You Have a Heart Problem or a New Joint

What is it?

Some heart problems make you more likely to get an infection in your heart. If you get a new joint, like a knee or hip joint, these areas can also get infected easily.

Did you know?

If you have a certain type of heart condition or a new joint, you have to be extra careful about infection. Germs in your mouth can travel through your blood to your heart, or to a joint. This can cause an infection in your heart or joint. To prevent this, you may need to take an **antibiotic** before going to the dentist.

What can I do at home?

- Tell your dentist if you have a heart problem, or if you have gotten a new joint in the last 2 years.
- Take the medicine exactly as your doctor or dentist tells you. You need to take the antibiotics one hour before your dental visit.

When do I call the dentist or clinic?

Call your dentist if your doctor says you have to take medicine before a dental visit.

Your dentist will work with your doctor to decide what is best for you. One of them will order an antibiotic. Tell your dentist if you are allergic to the antibiotic called **penicillin**.

If You Have a Heart Problem or a New Joint

What else should I know?

You may have to take medicine before your dental visit if:

- You have had **rheumatic heart disease**.
- You had a heart problem when you were a baby.
- You had a heart valve replaced.
- You had a joint replaced in the last 2 years.
- You have **mitral valve prolapse**.

The heart has flaps called **valves** that help pump the blood the right way. Mitral valve prolapse is a problem with these valves. The flaps are not working right. This lets the germs attach to them and make you very sick.

The antibiotic will prevent the germs from harming your heart or your joint.

Heart Disease and the Mouth

What is it?

Heart disease is when your heart is sick and doesn't work well. You can die if this happens.

Did you know?

Germs in your mouth can go through your blood to the rest of your body. This can happen if you have gum disease. This could hurt your heart.

What do I see?

You may not see anything until the gum disease is bad. Your gums may look red and puffy, or they may hurt. You may see your gums bleed when you brush or floss your teeth. (See page 22 to learn more about gum disease.)

What can I do at home?

- Tell your doctor if you have gum disease.
- Tell your dentist if you have a heart problem.
- Take care of your teeth to prevent gum disease:
  - Brush your teeth at least twice a day and floss your teeth every day. Use toothpaste with fluoride in it.
  - Tell the dentist if your mouth feels dry. Germs grow faster in a dry mouth. Ask the dentist what to use for a dry mouth.
  - Use mouth rinse or gel with fluoride to help prevent cavities.

When should I call the dentist?

Call the dentist if:

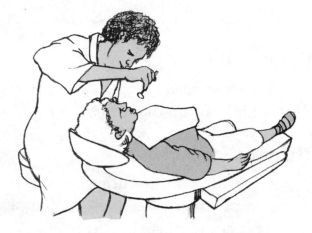

- your gums bleed when you brush or floss your teeth.

- your gums are puffy.

- your gums hurt.

Tell your dentist if you have a heart problem. This could affect your treatment.

See the dentist every 6 months for a checkup. The dentist will check for gum disease, and make sure your mouth is healthy.

What else should I know?

If you have bad gum disease, you may be more likely to have a heart attack. Be sure to tell your dentist if you have any type of heart problem before your visit. Tell your doctor if you have been told you have gum disease.

Word List

A

- **acid**—a strong liquid made by your body that can make holes in your teeth

- **adult teeth**—also called **permanent teeth**. These teeth form in the gums in children. They grow underneath the baby teeth and push them out when they are ready to come in. Most kids have all their adult teeth by about age 14. There are 32 adult teeth.

- **amalgam**—silver-colored filling, used to fill in cavities (holes) in teeth.

- **antibiotic**—a drug used to kill bacteria (germs) and cure infection.

- **appliance**—a device made by an orthodontist to correct a bad bite.

B

- **baby teeth**—the first teeth that babies get. These begin to grow in a baby's mouth at about 4 to 6 months of age. Most kids get all 20 baby teeth by the time they are 2 years old. These teeth are temporary. They start to fall out at age 5 or 6 and are replaced by adult teeth. Baby teeth are sometimes called **primary teeth** or **milk teeth**. They are very important.

- **bad bite**—when the teeth, lips, and jaw do not line up the way they should.

- **bite plate**—a thing made by a dentist that a person wears to stop them from grinding their teeth.

- **bone loss**—a loss of bone strength.

- **bottle rot**—when baby's front top teeth rot (decay). This happens when a baby drinks sweet liquids like milk from a bottle, and let them sit in the mouth.

- **bracket**—a part of braces.

- **bridge**—a set of one or more false teeth. It is used to replace missing teeth.

C

- **calcium**—a mineral that keeps teeth and bones strong. You can get it from certain foods.

- **canines**—teeth next to your front four teeth. Also called **fang teeth**.

- **carbohydrates**—a part of food that gives us energy.

- **cavity**—a hole in your tooth.

- **composite**—a mix of plastic and glass-like stuff used to make a filling.

- **crown**—a tooth-shaped cover for a broken tooth. Also, the part of the tooth that you can see above the gum.

- **cusp**—the raised surface on a back tooth.

D

- **dehydrated**—not enough water in the body.

- **dental cellulitis**—swelling in the mouth caused by infection. Dental cellulitis can spread to other parts of the body, like the head and neck. It is life threatening.

Word List

- **dental floss**—special string used to clean in between the teeth. Also called **floss**.
- **dental implant**—a metal post put into the bone under the gum with a false tooth on it.
- **denture**—a whole set of false teeth. There are upper and lower dentures.
- **diabetes**—a disease in which there is too much sugar in the blood.
- **diabetic**—a person with diabetes.
- **dry mouth**—not having enough saliva (spit) to keep the mouth wet.

E

- **erupt**—to break through the gum. When teeth come in, they erupt through the gum.

F

- **fat**—a part of food that gives us energy and is stored in our bodies to keep us warm.
- **fissured tongue**—a tongue that looks wrinkled or has deep and shallow grooves. This is harmless.
- **floss**—special string used to clean in between the teeth. Also called **dental floss**.
- **floss holder**—a plastic tool that holds the floss for you. It is sometimes called a **floss fork**.
- **floss threader**—a cleaning tool to use if you have a bridge.
- **flossing**—the process of using floss to clean the space in between teeth, and to clean the gums.

Word List

- **fluoride**—a mineral that helps stop cavities by making teeth stronger.
- **fluorosis**—white or brown spots on the adult teeth that form if a child gets too much fluoride.

G

- **gauze**—a very thin woven cloth used as a bandage.
- **geographic tongue**—a tongue that looks like the map of a country. It is harmless and goes away.
- **gingivitis**—red and puffy gums that bleed easily when there is too much plaque.
- **grooves**—long, narrow spaces on the surface of the tongue.
- **gum disease**—an infection (sickness) of the gums and bone that hold your teeth in place.
- gums—the pink part below your teeth.

H

- **herpes simplex**—a germ that can cause a sore on the skin. Also called a **cold sore** or **fever blister**.

I

- **impacted**—when teeth are stuck underneath the gums.
- **incisors**—your front eight teeth.
- **infection**—sickness caused by germs.

Word List

M

- **malnutrition**—when your body does not get the right nutrients. This happens if you do not eat enough healthy food. This can make you get sick more easily. Also, your body may not develop properly.

- **minerals**—certain parts of food that are important for your body to grow and be active. Calcium and fluoride are minerals.

- **molar**—a wide flat tooth in the back of the mouth. Molars are for mashing, crushing, and grinding food into smaller pieces. This help you swallow it.

- **mouth guard**—a soft plastic tray that fits over the top teeth. It helps protect them when you play sports.

- **mouthwash**—a liquid that helps wash the germs away when you swish it around in your mouth. Also called "rinse."

- **mouth sore**—also called an **abscess**. A painful, small bump that forms in the mouth. It's caused by an infection.

N

- **nerves**—thin fibers between your tooth and gum that let you feel hot, cold, or pain.

- **nutrients**—proteins, minerals, and vitamins. Nutrients are the parts of food that you need to stay strong and healthy

O

- **obese**—too heavy for your height.
- **obesity**—when a person has too much body fat.

- **oral surgeon**—a dentist trained to remove teeth and do surgery in the mouth.
- **orthodontist**—a dentist who is trained to fix crooked teeth, and get the teeth and jaws to line up right.

P

- **pacifier**—a rubber thing shaped like a nipple. Babies suck on this for comfort, instead of their thumb.
- **partial denture**—false teeth connected to a plastic base. You can take this out when you sleep or eat.
- **pericoronitis**—swelling of the gum over a tooth that is growing in.
- **permanent teeth—adult teeth**: the second set of teeth that replace the baby teeth.
- **plaque**—a sticky coating of germs on your teeth.
- **porcelain**—glass-like stuff used for crowns.
- **pregnancy**—the time when a baby is growing inside a woman.
- **pregnancy gingivitis**—a problem with your gums during pregnancy. The gums may get redder, hurt, look puffy or bleed.
- **pregnant**—when a woman has a baby growing inside of her.
- **primary teeth**—the first set of teeth. Sometimes called **baby teeth**. These teeth will fall out and permanent teeth will grow in to replace them.
- **protein**—a part of food to help build muscles.
- **pus**—a thick yellow or green liquid that comes out of an infection. It can smell bad.

Word List

R

- **retainer**—a plastic piece that you wear in your mouth to fix a bad bite.
- **root canal**—done by a dentist to clean and repair the nerve area of a tooth.

S

- **saliva**—liquid made in your mouth. Also called "spit."
- **sealant**—a plastic coating placed on teeth to help protect them from cavities.
- **secondhand smoke**—smoke coming from the end of a burning cigarette, pipe, or cigar. It is also the smoke that is blown out of the mouth of a smoker. You can breathe this in, even if you are not smoking.
- **six-year molars**—the biggest back teeth. These usually come in by the time a child is in first grade.
- **socket**—the hole where a tooth fits into the gum and bone.
- **space maintainer**—a thing that a dentist may put in your mouth if a baby tooth falls out too soon. It saves the space until the adult tooth is ready to grow in.
- **swelling**—puffiness.

T

- **tetanus**—a serious disease caused by germs getting into a cut. You get a shot to prevent tetanus.
- **tetracycline**—a drug that helps fight infection.

- **tongue**—the moveable muscle in the middle of your mouth. It helps you taste and swallow food, and also helps you speak.
- **tongue scraper**—a tool used to clean the top of your tongue. It looks like a small plastic rake.
- **tooth grinding**—squeezing and rubbing your teeth together, often when you sleep.
- **toothbrush**—a small brush with a long handle that you use to clean your teeth.
- **toothpaste**—gel or paste you put on your toothbrush to help remove the germs in your mouth and clean your teeth.

V

- **vitamins**—a part of food that is important for your body to grow and be active.
- **vomit**—throw up

W

- **wisdom teeth**—the third molars (18-year molars). They are the last adult teeth to come in at the back of your mouth. They usually come in between the ages of 17 and 21.

X

- **X-rays**—pictures of your teeth or bones.

What's in This Book from A to Z

What's in This Book from A to Z

What's in This Book from A to Z

People We Want to Thank

We wish to thank the following people for their help with this book:

Laura Arredondo
Albert E. Barnett, M.D.
Sheldon D. Benjamin, D.M.D.
Maria Cabrera
Emma Cannon
Sophie Cannon
W. Joseph Cannon, D.D.S.
Gina Capaldi
Judith Connell, Dr.P.H.
Jim Crall, D.D.S.
Justin Do, D.D.S.
Leticia Garcia
Maria Garcia
Liana Gergely
Talia Gergely
Kathleen Gibbons
Sandra Gonzalez
Stephanie Hoefer
Cynthia Holmberg, B.A.
Erika Jimenez, CNA
Gloria G. Mayer, R.N., Ed.D.
Carolyn D McLean, R.D.H.
Jorge H. Mestman, M.D.

Olga Montes
Alma Morales
Roseann Mulligan, D.D.S., M.S.
Steven A. Myers, D.D.S.
Elizabeth Ortega
Sandra Oviedo, A.A.
Alicia Pacheco, A.A.
Dolores Ramos, R.D.H.A.P., B.S.
Elvira Diane Rivas
Mirna Rivera
Ruth Sanchez
Donna Bell Sanders, M.P.H.
Gail E. Schupak, D.M.D.
Gail Strahs, D.D.S
Max Toledo
Michelle Upchurch
Michael Villaire
Carmen Villalobos
Carolyn Wendt
Shawn E. Wild, R.D.H., A.S.
Jackie Zazueta, B.S.
Christine T. Zwiebel, R.D.H.

Other Books in the Series

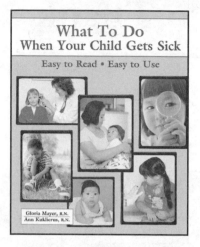

ISBN 978-0-9720148-8-5
$12.95

What To Do
When Your Child Gets Sick*

There are many things you can do at home for your child. At last, an easy to read, easy to use book written by two nurses who know. This book tells you:

- What to look for when your child is sick.
- When to call the doctor.
- How to take your child's temperature.
- What to do when your child has the flu.
- How to care for cuts and scrapes.
- What to feed your child when he or she is sick.
- How to stop the spread of infection.
- How to prevent accidents around your home.
- What to do in an emergency.

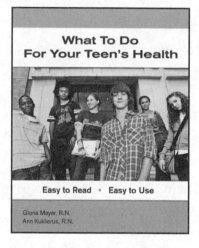

ISBN 978-0-9720148-9-2
$12.95

What To Do
For Teen Health

The teen years are hard on parents and teens. There are many things you can do to help your teen. At last, an easy to read, easy to use book written by two nurses. This book tells you:

- About the body changes that happen to teens.
- How to get ready for the teen years.
- How to talk with your teen.
- What you can do to feel closer to your teen.
- How to help your teen do well in school.
- All about dating and sex.
- How to keep your teen safe.
- The signs of trouble and where to go for help.

Also available in Spanish.
*Also available in Vietnamese, Chinese and Korean.
To order, call (800) 434-4633.

Other Books in the Series

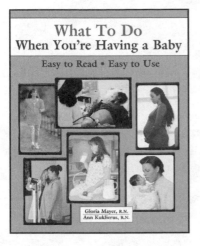

ISBN 978-0-9835976-0-5
$12.95

What To Do
When You're Having a Baby

There are many things a woman can do to have a healthy baby. Here's an easy to read, easy to use book written by two nurses that tells you:

- How to get ready for pregnancy.
- About the health care you need during pregnancy.
- Things you should not do when you are pregnant.
- How to take care of yourself so you have a healthy baby.
- Body changes you have each month.
- Simple things you can do to feel better.
- Warning signs of problems and what to do about them.
- All about labor and delivery.
- How to feed and care for your new baby.

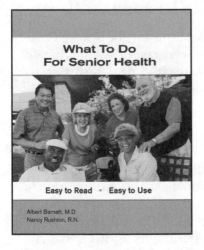

ISBN 978-0-9701245-4-8
$12.95

What To Do
For Senior Health*

There are many things that you can do to take charge of your health during your senior years. This book tells about:

- Body changes that come with aging.
- Common health problems of seniors.
- Things to consider about health insurance.
- How to choose a doctor and where to get health care.
- Buying and taking medicines.
- Simple things you can do to prevent falls and accidents.
- What you can do to stay healthy.

Also available in Spanish.
*Also available in Vietnamese.
To order, call (800) 434-4633.

Other Books in the Series

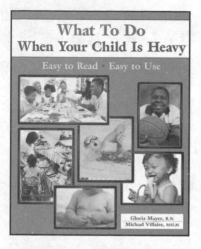

ISBN 978-0-9721048-4-7
$12.95

What To Do
When Your Child Is Heavy

There are many things you can do to help your heavy child live a healthy lifestyle. Here's an easy to read, easy to use book that tells you:

- How to tell if your child is heavy.
- How to shop and pay for healthy food.
- Dealing with your heavy child's feelings and self-esteem.
- How to read the Nutrition Facts Label.
- Healthy breakfasts, lunches and dinners.
- Correct portion sizes.
- Why exercise is so important.
- Tips for eating healthy when you eat out.
- Information on diabetes and other health problems of heavy children.

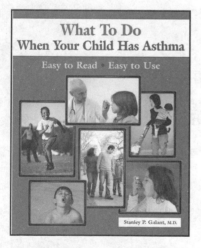

ISBN 978-0-9720148-6-1
$12.95

What To Do
When Your Child Has Asthma

Having a child with asthma can be scary. This easy to read, easy to use book tells you what you can do to help your child deal with asthma:

- How to tell if your child needs help right away.
- Signs that your child has asthma.
- Triggers for an asthma attack.
- Putting together an Asthma Action Plan.
- How to use a peak flow meter.
- The different kinds of asthma medicine.
- How to talk to your child's day care and teachers about your child's asthma.
- Making sure your child gets enough exercise.
- Helping your child to take their asthma medicine the right way.
- What to do for problems like upset stomach, hay fever and stuffy nose.

Also available in Spanish.
To order, call (800) 434-4633.